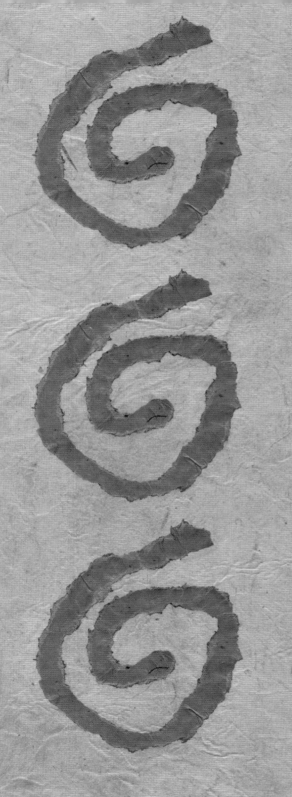

A Gift of Stories

Toby Adams, John, Susan Butler, Denise,
Susie Crooks, Pat Cumming, Lynda Delamore,
Graham Johnson, Julie Leibrich, Willie Lyden,
Kathryn McNeil, Robert Miller, Mary O'Hagan,
Sarah Pokoati, Patte Randal, Vince Reidy,
Jonathan Rodgers, Alasdair Russell,
Terry Stewart, Susan Tawhai and
Tessa Thompson tell their stories

gathered by Julie Leibrich

UNIVERSITY OF OTAGO PRESS/
MENTAL HEALTH COMMISSION

Published by University of Otago Press
PO Box 56/56 Union Street, Dunedin, New Zealand
Fax: 64 3 479 8385
Email: university.press@stonebow.otago.ac.nz

in association with the

Mental Health Commission

First published 1999
ISBN 1 877133 83 3
Reprinted 2000, 2006

Printed by Spectrum Print Ltd, Christchurch

Contents

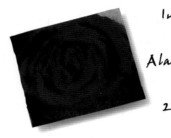

In Loving Memory
of
Alasdair James Russell

25 August 1953 –
13 February 1998

Introduction

When I was a little girl, my grandmother Gertrude used to tell me stories. On winter evenings we would snuggle up beside the fire and she would stare into the flames and gather up stories from the shapes of the burning coals. She'd look for dragons and fairies and strange faces, and listen to the hiss of the coal to find the words. As the heat of the fire grew, so the story grew, and if she lost its thread she would just poke at the fire a bit to get another chapter.

Sometimes the stories made me laugh, sometimes they made me cry, and sometimes they were scary. But always they fired my imagination and let me see new things, or old things in new ways. Sometimes she asked me to tell a story, too. At bedtime, as the flames subsided and the coals began to cool, the stories came to an end.

In this way, from my grandmother Gertrude, I learned a love of story, and decided to be a storyteller myself.

The Power of Stories

Stories have been told over the fire for centuries. Before written language was born, myths and legends were handed down by word of mouth in almost every culture. They were told in carvings and etched in pictures on the walls of caves, where they were added to and revised and kept safe in what were perhaps the earliest libraries of all.

Stories are one of the world's oldest and surest methods of teaching ideas. They help us *real*ise ideas: they make ideas real because they ask us to use our intellect and feelings at the same time, and sometimes they also speak to our spirit.

Personal stories, which tell us about individual experience, go one step further. They not only make ideas real, but they fill ideas with meaning. They show how a person tries to make sense of their world and they give 'the truth' as the storyteller sees it. They offer us people's wisdom.

Every story is unique – even if two people have shared an experience, they will tell different stories. This is not 'make-believe'. It is 'make-sense'.

Stories change and grow all the time. We continually revise our stories, not simply by adding new things that happen to us, but by reinterpreting the past in light of those things. It is as if we need to make sense of our lives in an ongoing way. Stories even change as they are being told – at that moment when they meet the listener – for as listeners, we add new meaning to them from our own experience.

This is why stories give us far more than information or knowledge. They give us an opportunity to understand something – to stand *under* knowledge – and the chance to gain insight – to see from *within*.

The Courage of Telling Personal Stories

We all have stories we could tell, but some of them we keep secret, locked inside ourselves for a very long time. Sometimes we are afraid to tell them in case people won't understand. Sometimes we have tried but nobody listened and the words got lost. Sometimes we are simply silenced.

Yet these are the kind of stories which can say the most significant things about life – even unlock the doors to life – but they take courage to tell. This is a book of such stories.

The stories here are by people who have, at some point in their lives, been diagnosed with a mental illness. In their stories, they talk about how they learned to deal with the illness and what they discovered about themselves in the process.

The act of telling stories can restore people ('re-store'). The telling of our story to someone who is genuinely interested and who relates to the telling through their own experiences is a very precious thing. But if a story is told and not understood, then a part of oneself has reached out into nothingness:

they died because words they had spoken
returned always homeless to them.
                    Janet Frame[1]

Some people even say when you lose your story, you lose yourself.[2]

It takes great courage to publish a personal story, for you have no idea who the reader will be, and cannot know if they are really listening. All these people have told their story before, but most have told it only to a few close friends. Very few have seen their story written down and put in a public place. The contributors here have found the additional courage to speak out about their experience in a world which is profoundly prejudiced against people with mental illness. This is one of the reasons why the stories told here are so precious.

Gathering and Presenting Personal Stories

A personal story belongs to the person who lives it, to nobody else, unless that person makes a gift of it. But it is often *other* people who tell stories about someone's experience of mental illness. These *other* stories are sometimes called 'case histories',

novels, newspaper articles.

The people in this book speak for themselves. Their stories were recorded on tape and written down in the teller's own words. I took great care to make sure that these stories are authentic, and that they belong to the people who told them to me. At the end of the book, I have given a detailed description of how I gathered and presented these stories. I hope you will take time to read it as it is very important to understand how context determines content in this kind of work.

The stories also speak for themselves. It was never my intention to comment on the stories or try to interpret them as I believe that this would be an intrusion on each person's integrity. This position led to my facing a dilemma as I came to the end of preparing the book for publication. Several people with whom I discussed my ideas about the book felt that I should summarise the stories. My training as a social scientist, and my background as a psychologist, almost tempted me to do this, for the material here is so rich. But I am glad to say that my instincts as a storyteller were finally stronger. All I am prepared to do is mention what *I* learnt as a result of doing this work, what insights *I* gained. And I have included these in my *own* story – for that is where they now belong.

The much more important ques-

tion is: What do the stories tell *you*? What insights will you get from reading them? Will you be able to open your minds and hearts and really listen? For this is a book of extraordinary gifts. To you. From people who want you to hear their story.

Understanding Mental Illness

In our society there is a vicious circle of fear and ignorance about mental illness: 'We fear what we do not know; and we do not want to know more about what we fear.'[3] There are so many obvious and overt unfair acts – the insulting images and language used about people with mental illness, the denial of their rights to good housing and employment, the fact that the mental health sector has had to fight tooth and nail for adequate funding.

Such things are not easy to deal with, but they are mostly visible and tangible, and can usually be pinned down and dealt with in the end. Much harder is the invisible, intangible prejudice, such as seeing mental illness as a person's primary characteristic, or even as their entire identity. This is what happens when we limit someone by a label. There is a danger we will limit them forever.

Some might say, for instance, this is a book by 'people who are mentally ill'. But I would say this is a book by people who have a lot of different talents and skills and achievements, *one of which* has been dealing with a mental illness that has significantly affected their lives.

Mental illness is not choosy; it affects people of all ages, backgrounds, abilities, and experiences. Some might say, this is a book by 'schizophrenics, manic-depressives' and so on'. But I say it is a book by people who are artists, mothers, fathers, typists, poets, lovers, researchers, analysts, doctors, sons, daughters, university teachers, sculptors, cousins, students, school teachers, reporters, gardeners, friends, health workers, factory workers, singers, voluntary community workers, cat-lovers, grandmothers, uncles, aunties, and sailors.

There is no one thing called 'mental illness'. Just like physical illnesses, there are many kinds, each of which differs in its effect on people's lives. Some illnesses are relatively mild, some extremely serious. Some people have a single episode of illness, some have episodes throughout their lives, and for others the illness is ongoing.

The diagnosis of mental illness is a complex matter. Even though there are standard criteria for diagnosis, not everyone would agree with the validity of this system, which tends to be categorical.[4] Some people prefer to describe mental illness in terms of the dimensions of human experience.

This book is about human experience rather than medical categories. That is why it does not give a glossary about specific diagnoses. Several of the people here were given more than one diagnosis over the course of time. Some accepted the diagnosis, some did not. Some found the diagnosis helpful, some did not. But most importantly, several explain how that diag-nosis became a label which became a problem in itself.

A diagnosis of mental illness does not say anything about a person's capabilities, personality, or future. The *vast* majority of people who have some kinds of mental illness: get better, can hold down jobs, make good partners, lovers, parents, and are not dangerous, and have a great deal to give to the world. In fact, the very act of dealing with a mental illness often gives people extraordinary strength of character.

Getting the right kind of help early on can make a great difference to the outcome. It can reduce the symptoms and speed up the process of getting well. Yet many people never seek help *at all*. Partly that is because the right kinds of services are not always available, but it is also because in a society prejudiced against people with a mental illness, it is very hard to 'admit' to having one.

The Mental Health Commission is committed to getting rid of the prejudice against mental illness that exists throughout our society – in communities, organisations, government, individuals, and in the health sector itself. One of the ways we can do this is to educate people about the reality of mental illness.

This book has been produced as part of the work of the Commission's Anti Discrimination Action Plan Team. It is one of the pathways on their journeys to end discrimination.[5] It is my hope that it will be a powerful resource – a source of inspiration for people with mental illness and those who are close to them, a special teaching tool for people who work in the mental health area, and a way of opening doors on mental illness and letting some light in, for *all* of us.

Julie Leibrich
Wellington, August 1999

Notes

1   *The Pocket Mirror* by Janet Frame. Vintage. 1992. From the poem 'The Suicides', p. 72.
2   Laurens van der Post makes this argument in several of his books, for instance, *The Heart of the Hunter*, Penguin, 1965.
3   Robert Miller, *Straight Talking about Mental Illness with emphasis on Schizophrenia.* Dunedin 1995, p. 15.
4   The most commonly used criteria in New Zealand are set out in the DSM-IV (the Diagnostic and Statistical Manual of Mental Disorders published by the American Psychiatric Association).
5   *A travel guide for people on the journeys towards equality, respect and rights for people who experience mental illness.* Mental Health Commission, Wellington, 1999.

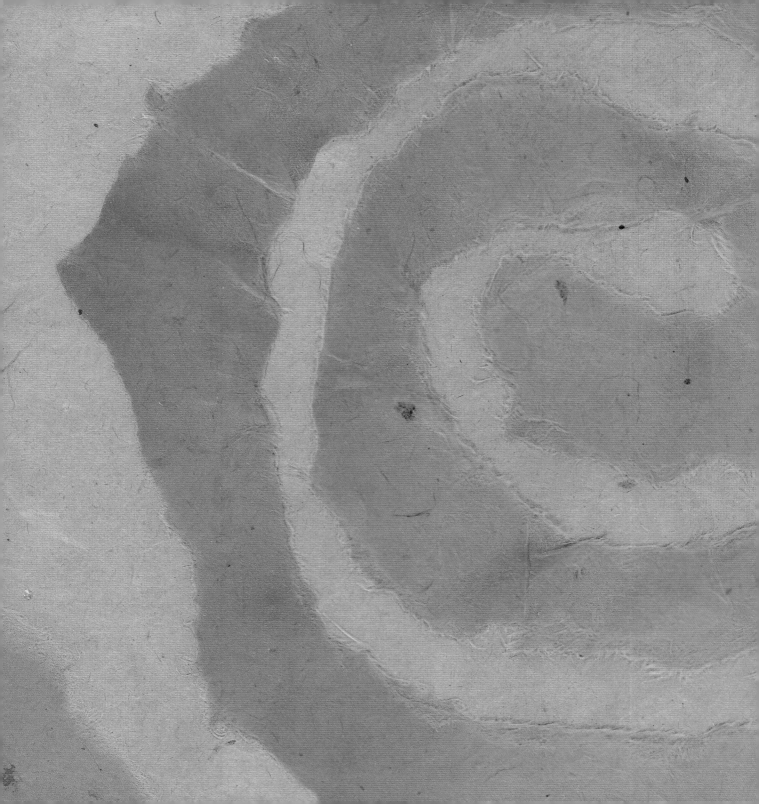

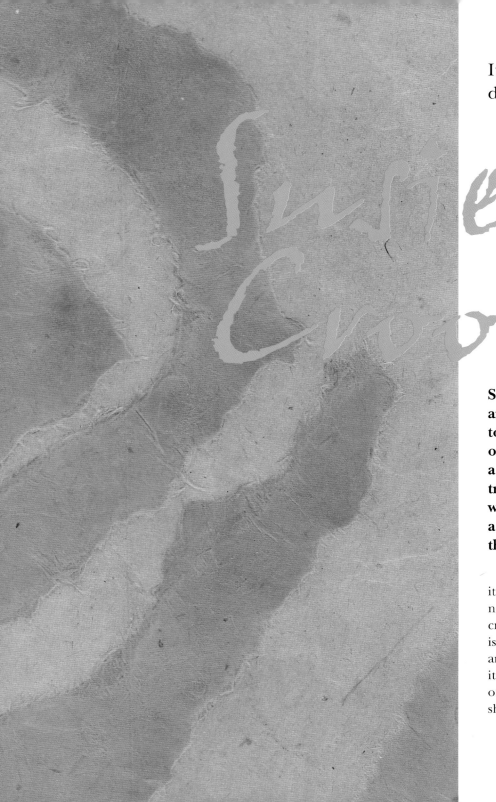

It's a privilege, not a disability, says

Susie Crooks

Susie is thirty-eight, an artist and fashion designer married to an orchardist. She is the co-ordinator of The Light House, a consumer-run resource centre in Hawke's Bay. She also works all over New Zealand as a staff training facilitator in the health system.

I've been wanting to write about it for a while because, to me, my illness is such a positive force – like my creativity and my brilliance as an artist come from that part of my mind, and it's a gift. That's how I project it. When I see crap on an *Assignment* or *Sixty Minutes* programme that shows mental illness as some sort of deviant, frightening, criminal illness, I think there's got to be people out there to counterbalance that view, because the only time that it was a disability for me was when I was in the medical model.[1]

I left home when I was fourteen and I got into sex, drugs, and rock and roll. In my paradigm it was not dysfunctional, it was exciting. I went to Sydney when I was fifteen and started having psychotic episodes, very similar to the experience of taking LSD, but I didn't need the drugs.[2] Because I was living in the Cross with a lot of drag queens and prostitutes and very colourful, tolerant people, I never got diagnosed, and I was accepted. I would just go off and they would just say, *Oh that's Susie going off.* I wouldn't sleep for a week. They looked after me but they didn't judge me.

Because of my family history, I rarely went to school. I never learnt to read or write. After every breakdown she had, my mother would shift the whole family, so we'd go to school here and there – but I wagged most of the time, anyway. She would have a breakdown about every three years, and we would change towns because of her wish to keep it secret.

I lived on the streets in Sydney. I was very well known for my graffiti. I wrote things like 'reel punks kant spel', and it got made into a postcard, and 'nukleyer war is hear to stay, mutate now and avord the rush', all spelt wrong. All over walls of flash buildings, multicoloured. I worked in the sex industry. When I was a kid in Sydney … everyone would go to bed at 1 o'clock in the morning ... I would take my cans of paint and trip out all over town, you know, graffiti.

I am a law-abiding citizen now – not that I ever got arrested. They could have traced me through my bad spelling! I supported myself, I was never on a benefit, and I couldn't read or write.

I was the life of the party. When I was high I could go all night, without drugs, just on my own natural stuff that I seemed to produce. I went to art school when I was sixteen, graduated with honours, got the top awards and opened up my own studio. I started exhibiting and stepped into a career.

By the time I was twenty-one I had been in all these major publications. I had exhibited at the NSW Gallery. I was lucky I had this gift. It was something that people wanted a bit of. My art was very appealing, you know – it was the sort of stuff people wanted. It's always been a joy.

Every few years I had a psychotic episode, but the shit really hit the fan when I was involved in a high court case down in Christchurch (I was a consultant expert witness) and I had a psychotic breakdown the week before the court case. I was sectioned into Sunnyside, and my mother, who I hadn't been close to for twenty years, flew down.[3] She transferred me to

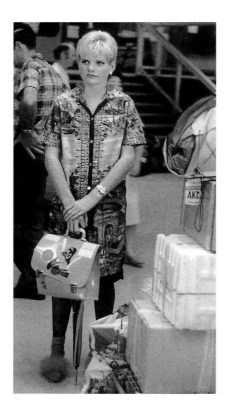

Leaving New Zealand when I was fifteen.

the psychiatric unit in Hawke's Bay, where I spent twelve weeks. The psychiatrist – he wasn't a doctor, he was a butcher. He was an old man, and he believed in totally medicating. He tried to treat me for being rude and obnoxious, when that is actually part of my personality and not something you can medicate out. I just had no respect for him, and so I lied to him and my section ran out and I got out.

I was on 30 ml of stelazine and 15 ml of something else – I don't know the name.[4] But the side effects from the high dosage gave me body tremors, and I felt like I was developing some sort of spastic condition – that's how high the dose was.

They wanted to put me on a six month order, and I managed, even though I was psychotic, to get my lawyer in.[5] The case was adjourned and I co-operated. I lied to staff and deliberately co-operated and got out, and stopped taking all the medication immediately.

I've had all sorts of experiences, I've worked in the sex industry, I've been raped. Nothing compared with the horror of this psychiatric unit. It was the most traumatic experience I've ever had. If you've ever read a Janet Frame novel, that's what it was like. It was just total madness, twenty-four hours a day, no privacy, all my personal belongings were stolen. I was sexually abused by another patient. I was assaulted. I had no safe space. They were trying to de-stim me in a very unsafe environment, and the fear and adrenaline that my body pumped through me just … They were trying to de-stim me using punishment.[6] They were putting me in seclusion. The streets of Kings Cross were safer than the psych unit.

It was unbelievable. I thought I had landed in a third-world country. I thought I was a criminal being punished. There was no humanity. The nurses were aggressive and rude. There was no safety. They showed no values, no respect; it was a totally dehumanising, humiliating experience, and because they had done urine tests and found that I was a marijuana-user they threatened my husband about getting the police if he didn't co-operate, so he was scared.

My mother also has schizophrenia and she has a long psychiatric history. They kept reminding me of that because they had treated her there themselves, and we've got the same name.

In the end I decided I would just behave myself like a good little child and lie to them and con them. I got out within a fortnight of making that decision. That proved to me they weren't interested in my well-being – they were interested in fitting me into a medical model that I didn't support. Seeing my mother go through it all, and I knew I had the illness – you

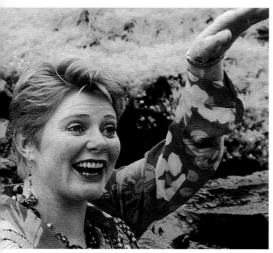

Photograph by Julie Leibrich

know, I hear the voices and all that.

Sure, I am permanently damaged, not by the illness but by the trauma of the treatment I received. I still haven't got over it. *I've* never had a problem with my illness.

In the crowd I mix with, eccentricity is quite acceptable. I still feel aggrieved, I still am going through a grieving process because being a psych patient I had no credibility. I was trying to tell people just how disgusting it was, and they would say, *No, that's your condition.*

I had had a huge company designer label I was exporting to the States, the UK and Australia, and I had over 200 piece-workers. I closed all that down and spent two years in recovery – not recovering from my illness, recovering from the, the, just the … I don't know what language I could use to describe my fear and the madness of the treatment. I just don't know what the words are. I can't think of them in the English language but it took me two years to just get back into mainstream life, you know.

Then two years ago I decided I needed to see a psychiatrist because I had another psychotic episode and I needed medication. It took fourteen days – even though my GP had written an urgent request – before I got access to a psychiatrist. I just had to take time off from work. I was under contract as a facilitator at the polytech at the time, and I had to take time out. Got the medication, got knocked out, recovered.

Since then whenever I'm going psychotic I see a psychiatrist. Usually after about three days of not sleeping, and I'm finding life hard to cope with. My mind's getting tired – you know, the racing – I want to switch off; I need to be knocked out. I go directly to the psychiatrist now, but that's been a battle … I have access to him now. This is the only service I use.

Now I take just 25 ml of melleril in the evening just to sleep, and a bit of stelazine if I'm PRM, if I'm having a stressful time. If I need it, I take extra melleril and stelazine and I take time out. I go into retreat, I go through a meditative process and I unwind. It's like my mind ties itself into a tight coil, and so I use alternative processes to unwind. Gardening, and resting. Not seeing anybody. I avoid people. I make sure that I'm in a very nurturing, caring environment. I'm very disciplined, I run my body like a sergeant-major. I get up at the same time. I make sure I eat. I make sure I go through the motions of living even if my mind is not engaged in it. So I fight. Yeah, I look after myself. And I see the psychiatrist as a tradesman, you know, that gives me tools; but psychiatrists are like hairdressers – each one gives you a different style, and if you've got a good one you're lucky.

After a psychotic episode I go through a period of black-dog depres-

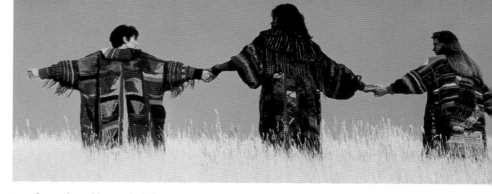

sion. In that state I'm very switched off. I get dulled and I need intellectual stimulation. I need to learn new things and expand my mind and get out of the thoughts. So I'll do courses – like I've just done a certificate in adult learning. Or I'll join a new group and my mind will be saying, *I hate it, I hate it, don't go, don't go, people are horrible,* and I'll go.

There's something in the relationship between humans that is a very healing process. I try to get out of my head, I try to be with people and get interested in their lives and quieten down my own stuff, so that I'm bigger than this stuff that's in my head – do you know what I mean? So there is something in the essence of communicating that is very vital. So that's what I do in the black dog depression. Sometimes it can last up to six months. I still make art but it's shit. Everything that I make is shit, but I still do it. I don't know when I'm coming out of it so I just keep going, and then one day the clouds clear. I take no medication for the depression. I just feel it's a natural process. It's like a rainy day – you know, like the weather.

I've got an excellent psychiatrist now. A friend, another psych patient, recommended this young man from England. He was a breath of fresh air

Above: My knitware designs. (Photograph by Nigel King.) Below: A poem I wrote.

There was a time when poeple thort the world was flat
When we foanld out it was rounld we looked out on a new herizon
Some poeple call my giff Maddness
dockdors nerds sykcriertrsets say I need help
I say they think the world is flat
I live in exstersee
I'v been to hell and back
my Jerny is far from strait
I can tell a good story
I live life to the full
I counld tie you in nots and titerlate your interlick
I have been harmed by main streem mederson
I fite for peace
The colourfull people agenst the grey people
I can never rest tell change takes place
Imbrace me like a new lover
I have much to offer

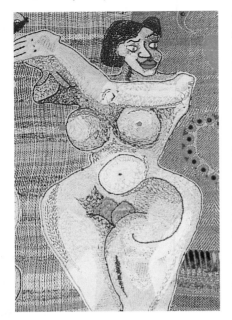

Detail from tapestry called Is it all right to be feminine.

that came into our service. He looks like a rock star. He's not a grey person. I went to see him and I just spewed out all my anger at the psychiatrists, and he accepted it. He did what I asked, he gave me the medication I was requiring. I had a breakthrough with him in the sense that I had found a liberal person within the system who actually respected my point of view. That was a breakthrough. He's rare.

The other psychiatrist was like God. He had sort of fascist nurses around him that, that punished, dominated and used power and control. Whereas the new head of the unit, Steve, he's made the staff go through retraining, workshops, he's sensitised the staff so there are improvements.

After being out of the system there was unfinished business. I had felt that I had been emotionally scarred and I couldn't get back into life until I had pursued this psychiatric diagnosis, because it had never been an issue for me. Prior to my diagnosis it had never been a disability.

It was as if I had changed my skin colour when I came out. I'm lucky because I am very cheeky and bolshie, and when I see someone baulk, or avoid the topic, then I get in there and say, *Look, it's an illness, you know – it's not a criminal offence.*

My admission was very public, in fact I actually had employees coming in to sort out business with me. I was still making decisions and running the business from inside the acute wing. But I still haven't really dealt with it in my profession as a polytech tutor; I haven't really shared with my associates. I'm not hiding – it's just not come up.

I don't want to see anyone else go through what I went through. I'm very angry, and I won't be satisfied until I see true change. I've always been very radical, I've been a member of Greenpeace and I've worked in prisons, I've worked on maraes. It's a gift, you know. I've always been an agitator, I've always been involved in protest movements, and I've got my teeth into this one, I want to see real change.

In my community, I'm accepted for who I am. I'm valued. I'm precious. But, you know, if you analyse my lifestyle you could say I was very dysfunctional. But to me I'm functioning. I live in ecstasy a lot of the time, which is something that people who haven't experienced it just can't imagine. I don't even mind depression, I just think, *Oh, I've got a headache* – it's not debilitating.

I don't see myself as sick. I mean, I hear voices and experience physical rushes and I have vivid dreams and fantasies. I hear nice voices, hilarious. Often very humorous, yeah. I have flashes and I paint them. They're brilliant. I often think that I'm writing my own movie, living in my own movie.

But I don't accept that it's schizophrenia – it's just a condition, it's just a facet of my personality.

I'm not an expert. I just know about myself. I think that if I channel my energy into the joy of life … The voices I heard when I was in the unit were like a living hell. I went into madness and lost my mind, but that is the only time that I have ever had a bad trip, you know. Vincent van Gogh. He's my hero because his inspirational madness came through in his paintings.

I don't do my fibre work commercially any more. After my breakdown, I just couldn't go back. So I'm into sculpture now, and ceramics. I've got my own studio and my own clientele and I make a living out of it. It's a lovely life, blissful actually. If I didn't have this gift, which is a precious gift, I would be just another grey person. I wish there were some way that people could know that it's actually a privilege to have this condition.

I'm lucky that my mother suffered from it because I was acclimatised to madness from a very young age. It was always in our house, my mother was always hearing voices and doing crazy things.

I just thought I was lucky. I never saw it as a handicap. Until I hit the wall with the medical model. Even the reading and writing was never a handicap. It's a privilege, it's not a disability. My second husband, he's an orchardist, and a very quiet gentle man who is not used to authority.

He's fantastic, he's fantastic. He's a man of few words. He's a gentle, loving man who works the land and just lets me be who I am. He has promised me that he will never let me go back there again. My father lives in the area too. They're my warriors, you know. When I go to the psychiatrist, if I'm psychotic and there's any risk of being sectioned, they'll come, and they won't let it happen. I'm never a danger to myself or others, so, you know, they're my shields.

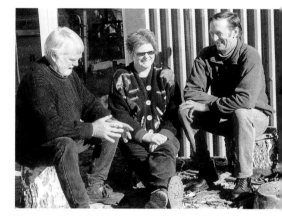

My two shields.

Postscript

Since the interview, I have become involved in the consumer movement nationally.[7] This has meant that I've discovered a whole network of people who, like me, want to raise the status of service users. It's been a privilege to meet so many fantastic and likeminded people.

People still want my artwork and so I paint on commission. And I'm just getting back into the fashion industry.

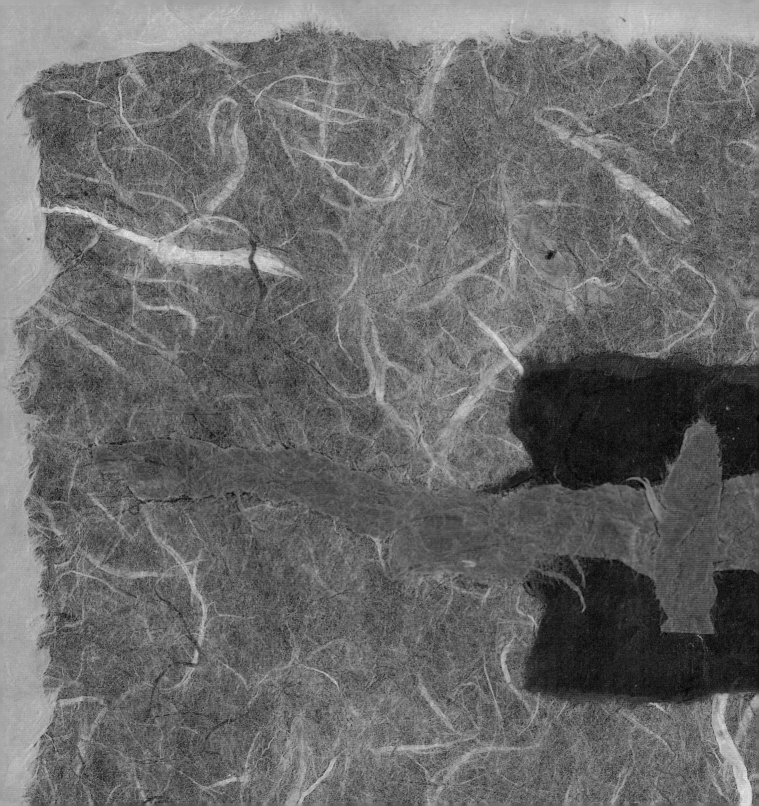

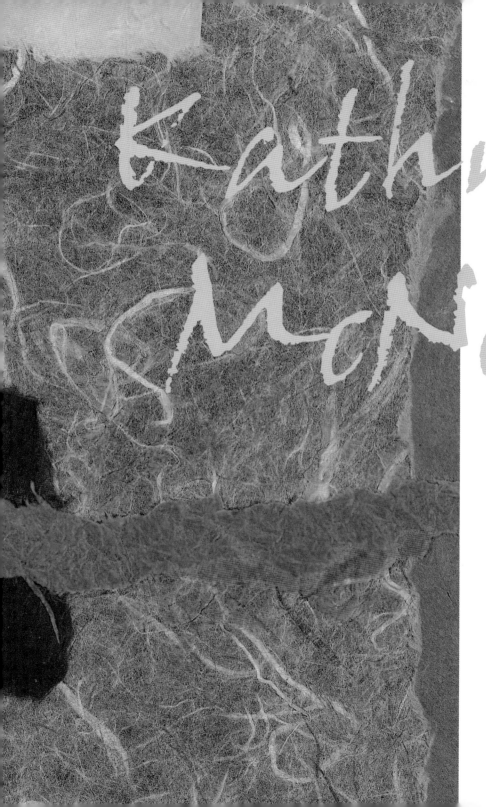

I just think it's about
being real, says

Kathryn McNeil

Kathryn is thirty-seven, a journalist living in Christchurch. She is the health reporter at *The Press*.

My periods of depression started when I was about nine and I was twenty-eight when I was diagnosed as having clinical depression.

My biggest fear was that I would get to a stage where I would not be able to work. Being alone was really bad. The idea of spending the day at home alone on the dole or sickness benefit … would have driven me to suicide, I think. I just couldn't bear my own company. I just couldn't stand it. I couldn't sleep, so I was awake all night. In the day I

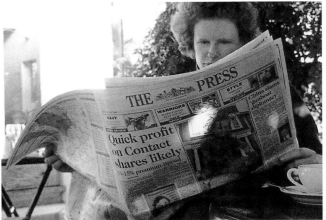

Reading The Press.

couldn't get myself going and I couldn't eat, didn't feel like eating anything. Nothing tasted good, everything felt dry in my mouth, though that was partly the medication I'd been put on.

It's very hard to identify a turning point. I think a willingness to accept the fact that I needed counselling was probably the big one. Especially the realisation that for counselling to work I had to co-operate. I had always survived in the past by keeping things to myself and not telling people how I felt or what was going on in my head. So that was a really scary thing for me to open up to somebody and tell them what was going on.

I have to say I did have quite a false start with the counsellors that I was going to. One was a psychiatric nurse out at Sunnyside.[1] We had a terrible personality conflict and it just was dreadful. That went on for about two years, and when I look at it now it was such a waste of time.

Fortunately I shifted away. I continued having counselling when I was living in Oamaru, but it was fairly low key. I also had private counselling in Dunedin on a regular basis, and that was better. When I came back to Christchurch I was put onto a very good GP and she did a lot a counselling sessions with me. She was talented, very gifted. I would have travelled to the end of New Zealand to keep going to her but she moved to Scotland and that was a bit far. I've got another GP now who's also very good.

But I think the turning point probably was being willing to talk it over with someone, and to get into the hard stuff. You know, the stuff I'd never ever talked to anybody about before. And finding the right medication was frustrating and soul destroying – persevering with medication when it wasn't working, trying another one when the last one didn't work, and trying another one when that one didn't work.

I feel the biggest barrier to making progress was a lack of continuity of care in the mental health system, until I insisted on seeing the consultant psychiatrist because I felt I was being shunted from pillar to post. I was fed up with seeing one registrar after another who had no idea of my history and had had no time to read my notes.

The consultant psychiatrist was very good and that certainly helped. I stuck with him for the next six years, and when he left the public sector I continued to pay to see him when I needed to.

I finally found the right medication, and I've been reasonably stable now for about three years. I keep taking my medication because every time I've tried to stop (with my doctor's help) things go wrong. First of all anxiety comes in, and then depression starts. I don't even notice it happening, but other people do and little subtle things in my life start to go wrong.

So I've learnt that the best thing is just to keep taking it. In a way that's quite devastating, because you do want to be medication free. But then, there are lots of people in the world who have to have medication for one thing or another. And it's just another one of those things. With me, it's just a chemical imbalance thing and once the drugs are out of my system then that imbalance recurs.

I used to not know I needed help until I was sitting in a crumpled heap at the bottom of the hill looking for the ambulance. But now, now I can feel it. So now I get about a quarter of the way down, and gathering momentum, before I get help.

I just have a sense that things aren't right. I guess I get more pessimistic about things. I get more lonely. I don't want to go out as much with people. Maybe I don't eat as well. Just little things. I don't feel in control. I just don't feel that I'm concentrating as well. Something isn't right. It's quite difficult to put a finger on what it is, but it's just something feels like it's starting to flip.

Then I go and see my GP and talk about it. Talk about how I'm feeling. We try and work out if there's a reason for it other than just the usual

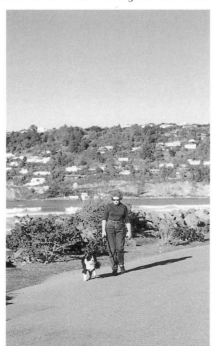

At Sumner with Zoe.

depression thing. And I usually feel a lot better after I've had a chat with her. Just talk about it, stay on the pills, get a bit of reassurance that it will come right again.

I'm sure there are a lot of GPs you can't talk to. I know there are. I mean there are GPs who just don't want to make the time commitment to deal with people who are depressed. They consider them 'the worried well'.

My GP listens and she's quite intuitive. She can tell. Even if I didn't tell her that I wasn't right, she'd probably know. I know her quite well now and I think she knows me quite well. My GP plays a big part. I know I can ring her any time if I need to, and I do have an after-hours number for her.

So I think people with depression need to find a doctor they can stick with, because often you don't know the signs yourself and you need someone else who can point them out to you. You know, *It seems to me you're a bit down* or, *You've only made negative comments the whole time you've been here, you haven't smiled once, you don't laugh, you haven't told me a joke, what's wrong?*

I used to give myself a hard time. But I don't now. I just say, *Oh well, here we go again.* You know, it's just like someone who has asthma. I guess they think, *Oh God, here we go again.* And there is nothing that you can really do about it except to try and keep yourself safe.

So I try to make sure I eat well. I try and keep working. And getting a puppy has been really good because it makes me exercise. Zoe's very good company. A dog's great for self-esteem too because you can only ever be half the person your dog thinks you are.

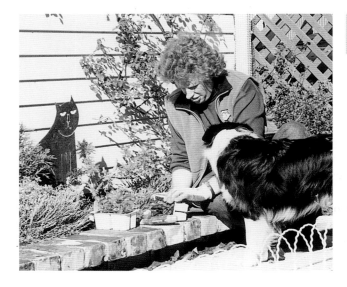

Gardening with Zoe and black cat.

With Zoe

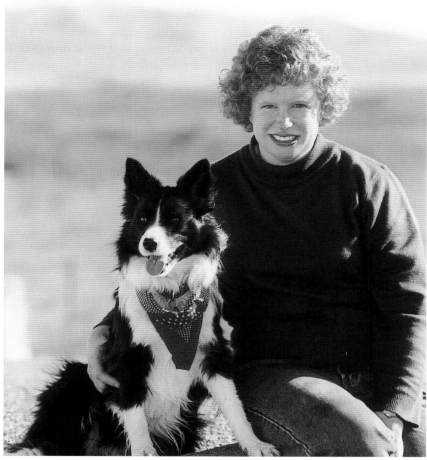

Photograph by Stacy Squires

Gardening's great, too. It switches your brain off. You don't have to talk to anyone, you don't have to concentrate. And you can take out any anger that you're feeling on your weeds, and your edges. I find if I'm feeling a bit low, by the end of a day's gardening, or even an hour in the garden, you feel, well you've achieved something. You've done something creative. You've been close to nature. And it's usually quite peaceful in the garden.

I like to meet friends and go out for coffee. I worked from home a lot in the last year and I found that's not a good thing for me to do because I get my energy from other people. So being able to go out to work matters. Earning money is quite important to me because it guarantees my independence.

I just think it's about being real. I think the other thing about keeping well is to be really honest about the depression. I don't hide it from any of my friends.

I talk to my friends. I'm very open with them about my depression. My friends understand it, and if they don't they just say, *Oh, I can't get my head round that at all.* Which is fine. There are people who don't understand why people get sick.

I don't talk to my parents about it very much because although I think they probably understand it quite well, I just don't feel comfortable talking to them about it. I don't really talk to family about it at all. I mean, they all ask but I just don't really care to share it with them. I think family are a bit close sometimes for those sorts of things. And if you feel a certain way, maybe your parents feel that it's their fault, even if it isn't.

I wrote an article about it in *The Press* in 1993 and five years later I still get stopped by people in the square who say, *You wrote that article on depression.* You know, I'm famously depressed!

The other thing that happened was that all these people came out of the woodwork at *The Press* saying, *Oh, I've got that too, you know,* or, *I've had a terrible time with depression,* and as soon as they say it you know that they have. But the other thing is, they don't front up, they won't own it. Even today they won't say that that's their problem. They just tell me privately. And they're terrified that the management will find out.

They told me they cut my article out and showed it to their family so that they might understand their depression better. I hadn't realised how much writing about me would help other people. I totally underestimated that. I wrote it because I was quite angry that people with depression are just pushed aside as being neurotic.

I don't see the point in not being real. It gets so complicated if you try

My kitten, Arnie.

to hide it. It's just part of life. Everybody gets depressed and there wouldn't be anybody in the world, I think, who by the time they die hasn't gone through a period of depression. And there's the whole couple of generations before us who went through terrible depression and never shared it, just bottled it up their whole lives.

I think until we really learn to be open about illness, whatever kind of disability it is that you have, or whatever condition, whether it's asthma, diabetes, high blood pressure, something that stops you from leading a normal life (and depression certainly does that), then we're not going to get anywhere. It's little problems like that that make you human. It's only Frankenstein and characters like that who don't get depression.

I've gained a lot more confidence. I know myself a lot better now than I ever used to and ever would have if I hadn't got depression. That's what the counselling has done. I feel really that having depression has been quite a privilege, and I thank it for a lot of things.

To me it was a blessing. I mean, I could have gone on in my life being the same old depressed insular little person that I was. But fortunately I got out of that. It's taught me a lot about life and other people and made me a much better person – a much stronger person too, because now I know myself emotionally.

Having suffering in your life is how you learn compassion. I think it's given me a greater understanding of where other people are coming from, and how they feel – that people can have problems, and that even if their problem seems really trivial, to *them* it isn't.

A lot of people who are depressed get into a real rut where they think there's nothing they can do about it. And won't even try. You know, *what's the point in trying?* And that's a very depressed person's view of things.

The big question I used to ask myself when I was really depressed is *What is the purpose of my life? Why am I here?* And I hated being here. I thought, *What's the point? Why am I here? I might as well not be here.* Then one day it dawned on me: *there isn't any point. So you might as well stop looking for one.* Once you stop looking for the point, things get a whole lot easier.

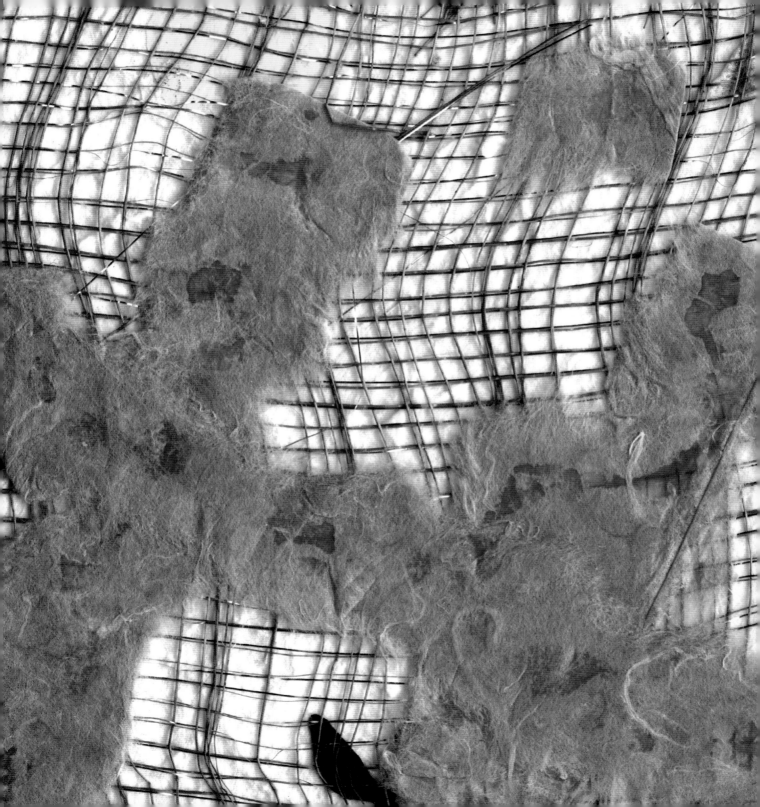

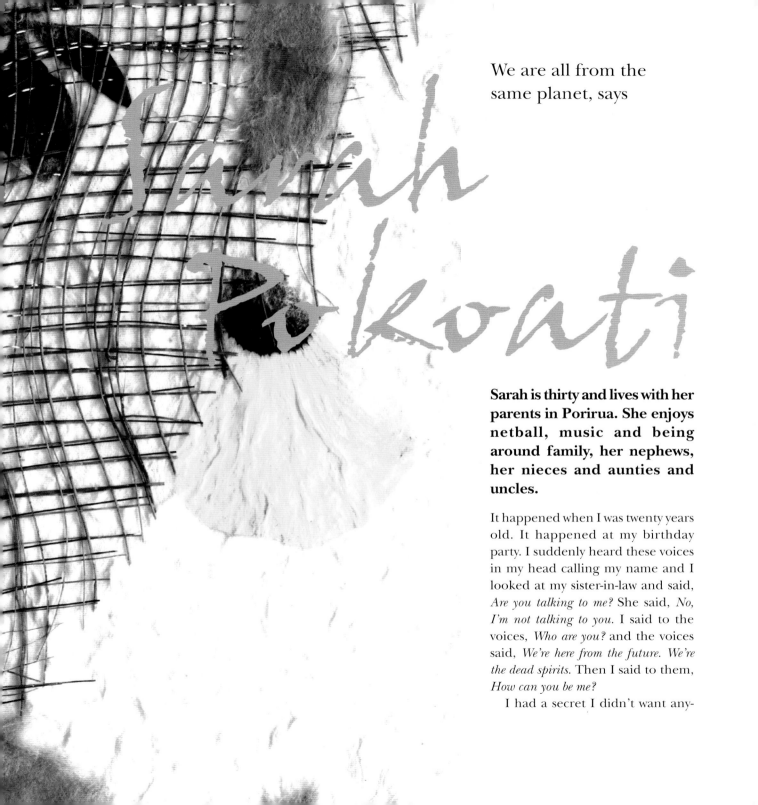

We are all from the
same planet, says

Sarah Pokoati

Sarah is thirty and lives with her parents in Porirua. She enjoys netball, music and being around family, her nephews, her nieces and aunties and uncles.

It happened when I was twenty years old. It happened at my birthday party. I suddenly heard these voices in my head calling my name and I looked at my sister-in-law and said, *Are you talking to me?* She said, *No, I'm not talking to you.* I said to the voices, *Who are you?* and the voices said, *We're here from the future. We're the dead spirits.* Then I said to them, *How can you be me?*

I had a secret I didn't want anyone to know, and only I knew that I had it. They asked me to tell them my secret, so I knew they *must* be me. They said they were testing me for the future, to see if I could reach my goals in the future.

It wasn't until a couple of days later that I could hear the voices all the time. I asked them their names, but they said they were my dead spirit from the future. They had come back in time. They were talking about my future. They said I was going to be a netball player and that I was going to be a model too and an actress and a singer. But I didn't really believe them because of my weight. I thought it couldn't be true.

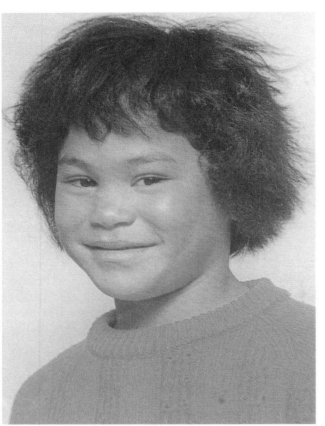

Me at five years old.

I didn't want to tell my parents about it because I had watched a lot of programmes like 'Sybil', the woman with mental illness.[1] I kept it to myself because I didn't want to go to a nut-house. After watching that programme I thought, *Oh no, I don't want to go to that place, everyone will think I'm crazy.*

So I went to Australia and my sister took me to a doctor who asked me if I heard voices, and I said I did. He said he would keep it confidential, but he didn't. He told my sister and I didn't like that. I didn't want anybody to know that I was schizophrenic (that was how they explained it to me). I felt embarrassed. I thought, *I'm the only one in the world.* I was really embarrassed. I didn't like the idea of her seeing that I was a schizophrenic after watching that programme 'Sybil'.

After that my sister and I got into a fight and she rang the police and they took me down to the police station. I cooled down for a while and they didn't press any charges. When I saw the police I thought, *Oh I may as well go before there is any trouble.* So they took me to this place called Cumberland Hospital for the mentally ill.[2] This was in Australia.

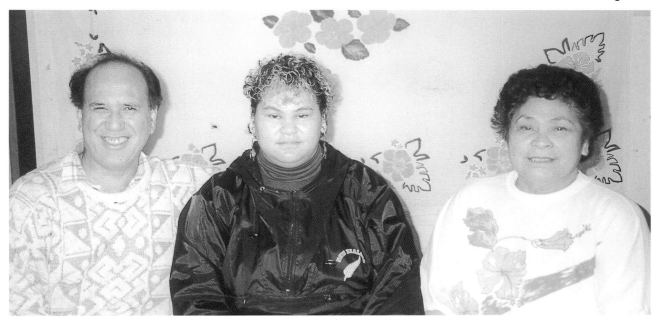

Me with Mum and Uncle Sam.

I said to them, *How long am I staying here for?* The doctor said for one night. But when the next day came I saw my sister and she had my pyjamas and that in the bag. That meant I was staying even longer. I felt really really angry because I felt the doctor had lied to me. I was really angry and when she came I tried to attack her. I said I didn't want to see her and so she went away. I was there for about six weeks, I think. I was twenty-one.

I've been in hospital about three times in all, but not since 1996. That was the last time. When I was in hospital I found all the Pakeha nurses used to treat their race better.[3] We were looked at like underdogs. Like they always got their dinners served first. They got special privileges. Us Islanders didn't. We were just chucked in there, had breakfast, lunch, and tea and that's about all. But I haven't been in there since 1996, so they might have changed.

Schizophrenia has changed my life. When I wasn't schizophrenic I used to always go out to nightclubs with my cousins and go to parties, but when I became sick I pulled away. I didn't want to be with them, I just wanted to be with myself. I excluded myself from everybody because I thought, *they are not like me and they won't understand.* They will talk about me and laugh.

Especially when I came back from Australia. Everybody was very ignorant. They said, *You shouldn't be drinking; the doctor said you're not allowed to drink,* and I said, *Well, the doctor said I can have a few, that's all right, I know when to stop.* I don't like other people telling me what I should do and what I shouldn't do, because I'm old enough. I was twenty-six and I said to them, *I'm old enough.*

But people watch TV and listen to all this stuff on the news which says that everybody with mental illness is in the same boat. As if we all do everything together. We all have our mood swings, but people act differently towards schizophrenia.

I think Islanders think it only happens to Pakeha, it doesn't happen to us. When it does happen they say, *Oh Christ, she's a nutter.* Cook Islanders are very ignorant. They think you're crazy. *You belong in a nut-house, you don't belong to us. You should be with people that are like you.*

But a lot of people in my family suffer mental illness. It's hereditary, in the genes. When I came back from Australia, I found out that a lot of my family had the same mental illness and that made me happy, thinking I'm not the only one in the family.

My parents were very helpful. My mother was there through the whole thing and my father, too. But I lost a lot of my friends when I became sick. I just excluded myself and I didn't want to be around them.

I've always been very quiet and I'm a very gentle person, really. Most of my cousins think I'm like a teddy bear! But when I became ill, it changed my whole personality. When I became sick, I became very very violent.

I think the worst time was when I hit my mother. The voices tried telling me that she wasn't my mother, that somebody had taken her place. So when she came back from shopping, I attacked her. Another time, I got into a big fight at one of the mental institutions in Sydney. I was put in solitary.

I'm not like that any more. Now, I've settled down. I feel more calm, more relaxed and I don't feel that the world is against me any more.

I tried to commit suicide several times. I would take a whole lot of pills. If I got upset, I used to take an overdose. But now I'll never do it again.

The medication they've put me on made a big difference – clozapine. It was like a miracle. I've been on it since 1996 – for three years – and it has hardly any side-effects. I think it's a miracle drug. Even my family reckon it's a miracle because it's really healed me. My family understand now. They've seen the difference between what I was before and what I'm like now. I'm getting

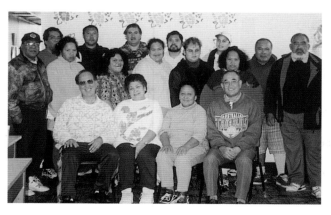

Tamarangi Group, Porirua, 1999.

there. I'm getting better. I've got to be really patient. I've had no suicide attempts, I have no grudges, I'm not violent, and I'm very patient.

I take my medication now. When I was on other medications, I used to flush them down the toilet. But this one I don't mind taking! I remember every night. I know it is doing something good for me and that's why I take it. I see a psychiatrist every month and get my prescription. We talk about how I am, and I can tell them I'm fine.

Also I come here to the Tamarangi Group, which is about family and means Children of God.[4] It is a good place if you want to get together with family. We all are related to each other. Some of us are cousins, some of us are uncles or aunties. It is a Rarotongan group. Sam's our leader. We sing and do arts and crafts. We go off on picnics and have barbeques if the weather is hot. It's sociable. But if we have a problem we all talk about it. If someone's having a bad day Sam takes them off and talks to them in a room. And when they've settled down, they come back to the group.

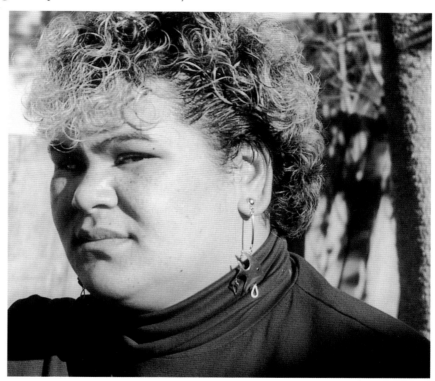

Photograph by Julie Leibrich

I'm starting to go out more, mix with people. I feel much happier because I can see everybody in my family and I've got cousins who really like me. I'm much happier with my life now, *much* happier.

I go out once in a while with my cousins. I like to sing Rhythm and Blues. I sing around home. I like all black music and some white music, too. My favourite is Boyz-to-men.

I'm doing a training course called Modern Age, run by Social Welfare. You do administration, computers, and clerical work. It's to help you get back into the workforce. I go every day from nine to three and I'm hoping for employment at the end of it.

I'm also being helped by Focus Trust, who try and find employment for people with disabilities. I find I've been knocked back on some of my inter-

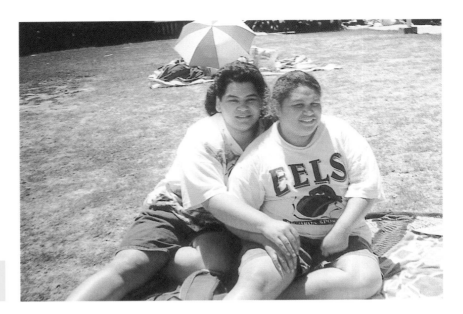

With my niece, Christine, 1997.

views because of my mental illness. There were a couple of jobs I applied for and never got, although I was qualified for them. I've got a CV which shows the jobs I had before I was ill and it shows my educational qualifications. I think the boss was prejudiced because I have schizophrenia.

One thing I don't like is how people called you 'schizo' for short. I don't like that. I think it's degrading. It's like someone in prison, like calling them a convict. They don't like that and I don't like being called a 'schizo'. We all have our own virtues in life.

I live with my parents. I am the youngest of nine. I'm the baby of the family. I've got five brothers and three sisters. I wouldn't want to live anywhere else because I like to be home where I can do what I want.

I've lived with my parents all my life. Well, you don't want to be on your own all the time. When you're sick and unhappy you always depend on your family to be there for you. They *are* there for me now. They have watched the difference. Now, they encourage me to get better. They used to limit me in doing things but now they are all right. I was a real basket case. I reckon I was crazy then. I wouldn't admit it before but now I think I was.

I really feel sad about the past. I really feel sad especially about the way I attacked my own mother. My mother, my brother – I attacked them with knives. I really feel bad. It upsets me when I think about it. But they have forgiven me. They have been really good to me. They just turned a blind eye. My mother used to go to schizophrenia seminars with me in Australia, and she comes to Tamarangi Group too and helps Uncle Sam. It's good to have her around. Love can heal schizophrenia.

I used to think, *Oh, nobody wants me because I'm crazy.* Nobody used to listen to me. Usually, I like to keep to myself, I like my own secrets. But I am talking to you because I want to help people. A lot of people with schizophrenia feel lonely. I want all the people with schizophrenia to know that they are not alone. There are people who have been in the same boat. I want them to *know* that they are not alone. I want to say to people: *Just have faith in yourself. Don't isolate yourself in the world. You are not the only one.*

I used to be really religious. I used to go to Sunday school, to church with my parents, but I have lost my faith in God since I became sick. I blame Him because everybody says He has the power to heal. I think *why can't He heal me?* I've had schizophrenia for ten years. If He can heal people who are blind, then He can heal people with schizophrenia. I told Uncle Sam about this, and he has said if that's your belief then that's your belief. One day I might believe again.

I'd just like to be healed. I'd just like to have a normal life. Go on and do things that I want to do. Not being classed as schizophrenic any more, but as a human being like everybody else. I'm not an alien. We are not aliens, we are human beings. Just because some of us have a mental illness and some don't, we are *all* still human beings. We are all from the same planet.

I still have dreams. Well, I didn't really want to be a netball player! I believe in having a happy life: good family, friends, entertainment, hobbies. I want to get married and have a family one day. I'm thirty. I'm not getting any younger. I'd better go out in the water. I better try and find some fish!

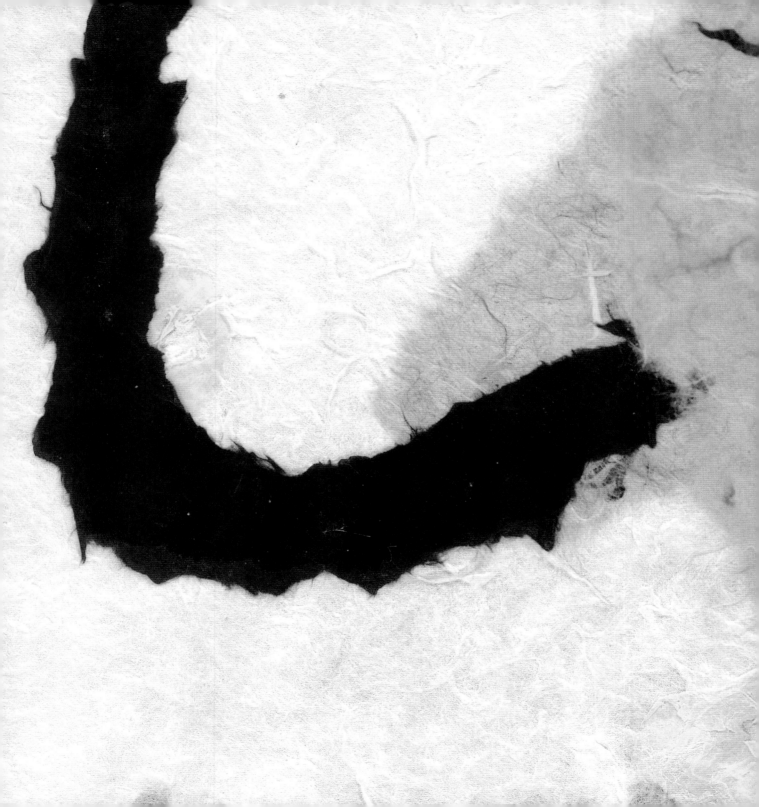

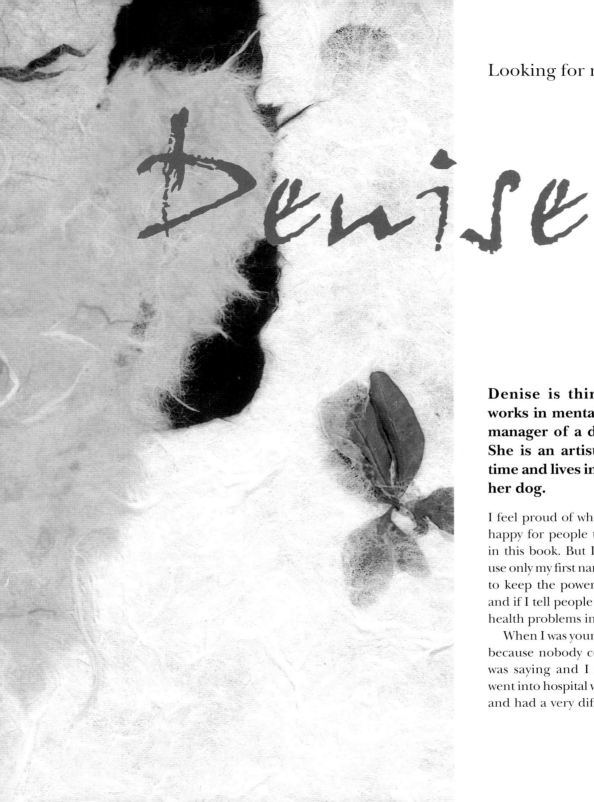

Looking for my self, says

Denise

Denise is thirty-three and works in mental health as co-manager of a drop-in centre. She is an artist in her spare time and lives in Dunedin with her dog.

I feel proud of who I am, and I am happy for people to know my story in this book. But I have decided to use only my first name because I want to keep the power to choose when and if I tell people about my mental health problems in the future.

When I was younger I was suicidal because nobody could hear what I was saying and I felt desperate. I went into hospital when I was sixteen and had a very difficult experience

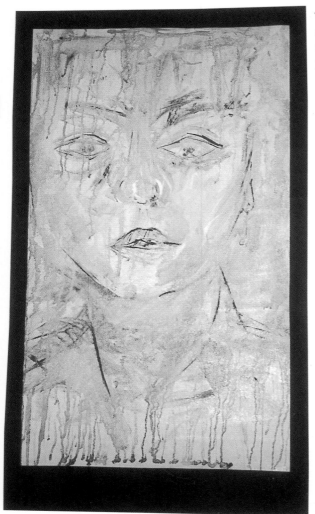

with all sorts of diagnoses and all sorts of medication. Right through my school years and adolescence I was being referred to psychiatrists. So it was always there. And I had severe behavioural problems at school.

I asked for help in every way that I could. When I had nowhere else to turn, suicide was my best option because I just couldn't tolerate the feelings I had. It wasn't that I actually wanted to die, but after I had been in the public health system, my spirit was broken. It changed to the point where I *wanted* to die and that was very different for me.

Then I left home and refused to have anything to do with the mental health system because of how I had been treated.

I had problems on and off over the next ten years, but managed to hide them. I felt I needed to hide them from my work, from whatever. I would go away for six months but manage to stay on the job roster so it didn't look like there were gaps in my CV. Somehow I could cover them up.

But about four or five years ago, after a break-up in a relationship, I became very unwell and I asked for help, quite directly. I knew that I was depressed, but I was refused the help that I needed. So I responded by becoming more bizarre in my behaviours and communicating indirectly in any way that I could so that people would listen. I had a sense that what I did didn't actually matter – like I could do quite the most outrageous things and it made no difference.

This was how I came into the public health system again, and it was a total disaster. A total, total disaster. I was totally out of control and I had practically starved myself to death. These were all ways of communicating that there was something terribly wrong. They were unconscious and indirect ways of asking for help but eventually they got me the attention I needed. My thoughts were becoming quite dangerous and I was committed to Kingseat Hospital.[1]

I was in and out of Kingseat until, at one committal hearing, a judge heard that I wanted counselling, not more drugs, and ordered the hospital staff to support me in this.[2] I went briefly to Kahanui Village but I was much too unwell for their programme and had to leave.[3] I was frightened and desperate and in the process of getting home I assaulted a mental health staff member after she had yelled at me and told me I was stupid.

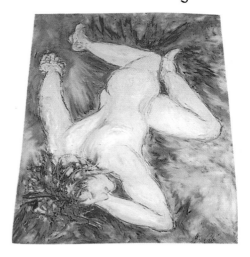

They committed me to Tokonui, and that was the worst, worst, worst thing.[4] For a start I was taken straight into an isolation unit, and I was strapped down until I was in a side room. Of course we were going through the rigmarole of having to strip naked – and if you don't do it, they'll do it for you sort-of-thing – and not being allowed to be left with your knickers or your socks or anything like that, and being left in this place.

Nobody came to speak to me for ages. There was some interesting graffiti on the wall like 'Motel Hell', or something like that, and I thought afterwards, that's not wrong.

I was trying to talk. I asked to see a patient advocate and they said, *Sure, you can ring one*, and I said, *Where's the phone?* and they said, *You're not using our phone, you can use your own.* I said, *I would like to see a district inspector*, and was told, *Yeah okay.* Then I said, *I'd like to see a doctor* because I had quite a serious cut on my leg and it was going septic. I ended up having to scoop the pus out of it with a plastic spoon they gave me to eat with, because they didn't let me see the doctor. But if you read the notes now, they said that I refused to see a doctor – they did. I just broke down and cried. I said to them, *Look, you're breaching all my rights here, I know what they are.* And they said, *No, we're not.* I would say, *Why are you keeping me in isolation?* And they'd say, *You're not in isolation – there's just no other people around for you to be with.* That was a lie.

After a few days I managed to get out of isolation, into the main ward. In the main ward, we were locked into the dorms. There was a woman lying there in full light – there was a light outside all the windows so you couldn't get any darkness or peace at night, but this woman was lying there masturbating, which was quite frightening for me at that stage. There were no doors on the toilets, and the men and women used the same area at times. Everybody had to have showers at the same time, so they'd use one shower, and all the women would go in, and then all the men would go in. I felt very unsafe that there were no doors on the toilets. I certainly didn't want to go into the toilet. They shepherded people from one room to another so that everybody was in the same place at the same time.

You had to go outside for three hours at a time, if that's what they wanted you to do, whether it was raining or whatever. There was a ten-foot wire fence enclosing the ward and a recreation area. We were caged in. You couldn't sit down and watch TV or read a book. There was nothing to read in the ward. When we were locked all together in the lounge area, there was a women's toilet in the lounge, but there was no lock on the door. It could open and you were just sitting there on the toilet in front of a whole room of men and women. And I had no access to any of my own clothes.

Woman with a difference.
This is the picture that I had on the front of the invitations to my exhibition in August 1998, an exhibition portraying a consumer's experience of using New Zealand mental health services.
This picture is a comparison between the art I did in art therapy and art I did for myself. It shows the changes in myself.

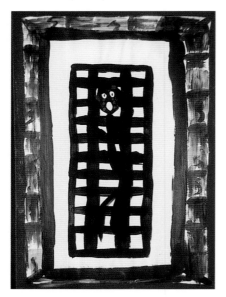

Above: **Prison**. This is what's on the inside and what's on the outside. Lots of bright colours on the outside, nobody can actually tell, and on the inside just trapped, screaming like.

Right: When first in Ashburn Hall (not in art therapy) I was just painting on my own in the art room. I was learning to express myself through art as my most effective form of communication.

When I was in an isolation lounge, there was this one guy that I could see through a glass door and he could see me. He was drooling, he was tied in a straitjacket; this is only four years ago, he was in a straitjacket. He was drooling – so drugged he could hardly move. And we both just sort of reached out. There was a real connection, like people that were being tortured.

The other thing that really freaked me out was this fire alarm went off and all the nurses disappeared to see what it was. I was locked in a room for about ten minutes with the whole window covered in smoke. I had no way of getting out. That was incredibly frightening.

It's taken me a long time to talk about it to a point where I can say a lot of what happened. It was really that the staff were so abusive and I was totally under their control. There was nothing that I could have done. Unless you have ever had that experience you could never, ever convey what it felt like. The powerlessness. The abuse. I was only in Tokonui for five days, but during that time my spirit was broken. I went back to Kingseat for another eight months while I waited to be transferred to Ashburn Hall.[5]

The first time I began to receive appropriate treatment and started to recover was when I got to Ashburn Hall. This is also where my art work starts. The first process that was helpful in my recovery is reflected in my

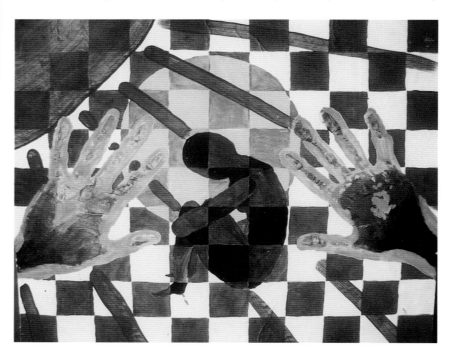

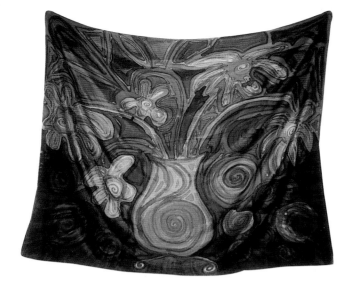

Handpainted silk scarf.

art therapy. It was the beginning steps. After that first art therapy session, I just wanted to paint. I wanted to get it down. I wanted to get it out. I wanted to explain what was going on.

When I did that art therapy at Ashburn Hall I thought, *Yay, at last I can actually express what's going on*, but I was actually told I couldn't express my homicidal feelings there because it was frightening for other people. This was the first time I began to realise that what I said and did actually had an impact on other people. This was a new concept for me.

I want to make clear that I don't think that naturally I am a homicidal person. But I got to the stage where I was beyond caring, really. Like I felt like nothing I did made any difference, and nothing that I said made any difference. So *what the fuck* sort of thing.

I was at the hospital for six months but I really pushed people over the limit all the time. I was quite violent at times, and I had to leave. One of the things that I needed to learn was to get a sense of my own boundaries and to get a sense of other people's boundaries.

I continued seeing my therapist and that was really important for my treatment and my recovery. After a further six months I was allowed back into the programme. I continued to see my therapist through that time, and after I left. Ashburn Hall never gave up on me.

I guess if I had to sum my recovery up it would be *having enough awareness to make choices for myself.*

With the personality disorder I had, there were a lot of parts of my personality which hadn't developed, that other people take for granted. For a start, I had no empathy. I didn't know that I didn't have empathy, because I actually cared about people – but really I had no empathy. I had no under-

To Tim

You've reached out your hand in a fatherly way
And you've touched deep inside but I know I can't stay.
It pains me to think that the end's drawing near,
Our closeness will die but I know you still care
As you've done from day one though I didn't quite trust
That to help me be free to love first you must
Cause pain in my heart as has happened once before
Though never quite healed, now opening a door
To a world worth exploring, do I dare risk a look
For already I've feared and in fear I have shook
As a cold chilling wind has flowed bitter through my veins
Deep inside though I'm healing I still feel the old pains
In my anger I have spat on the graves of the old
As a deathly poison seeps to the depth of my soul.
But something of you and the time we have had
Has softened my heart. Deep inside I feel sad
For the things that I've seen and the things I have done.
I know I have hurt but to this I was numb
You have planted a seed and from this love has grown
Both for you and for others in a way once not known.
My branches reach more strongly as our time starts to perish
But the gifts you have given I'll remember and I'll cherish.

standing of concepts coming from other people's points of view whatsoever.

The point of psychotherapy has been having a relationship that's worked, that's not abusive, and that's really consistent. The thing that has been the most important really is having the consistency of the relationship. There have been boundaries, and I have learnt about that. I have learnt to acknowledge that there are two people in the relationship and that there is stuff going on from both angles.

One problem that I have is poor impulse control. Before, if somebody had pissed me off, I would have whacked them. I just had no concept that what I did actually had any effect on anybody.

Now I do have that awareness. That developed from being in Ashburn Hall with other people. I was in groups where people were saying, *Well, this is what you have done and this is how it has affected me.* It helped me to develop an understanding of what I did. So now if somebody pisses me off, I have much greater choice of what I can do.

To know that I can actually live through the ending of the relationship is important because my depression is very tied up with loss, which is very tied up with death.

I am on permanent medication, so I don't have the real depression that I had, although that still comes and goes. It is not only that my moods don't swing as much, but I have also learnt to control them. I recognise the signs when I am getting too stressed. I just can't take it for granted that I will never become unwell.

Another really important part of my recovery, apart from the personal growth through the psychotherapy, has been development of my spirituality. I belong to the spiritualist church. It's been very helpful because I've had so many people close to me die that I needed to form my own ideas and beliefs about what I believed in before I came to die. The psychotherapy helped me develop my self-awareness and allowed me to make choices, but a spiritual awareness has developed a softness in me

I work in mental health now, in a drop-in centre, and that was a big decision to make because I didn't like the idea of becoming a service provider. One of the reasons I have really dedicated my life to making a difference to people's experience when they have a psychiatric disability is that I take it very, very seriously. I have had so many people, so many friends, die. So many people I have known have lost their life, haven't made it. I consider myself very, very lucky.

I make a conscious choice now to become more politically aware, and more educated, to do what I can do. I am very grateful for my self-awareness. I still have a lot of feelings and sometimes it's a real struggle to keep going. I don't know if I will ever recover fully.

I am still a raw person. I am really aware that I've got a long way to go. I've got a lot to learn, and that's both in my personal life and my art work.

I believe quite strongly that we don't necessarily have any control over the events that happen in our life, particularly when we are younger, but I do believe that we have a choice in how we respond to what has happened. And the only way we have that freedom of choice is by having a consciousness. That's what psychotherapy and recovery has meant to me. Developing the consciousness so I can actually choose how I respond to situations that I find myself in.

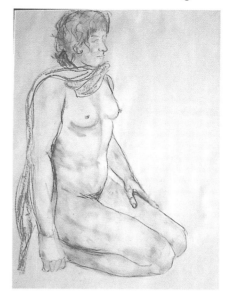

Woman in the scarf. Life drawing sketch, once again showing the changes going on inside myself.

Some of my biggest problems were how little I valued myself, and I struggle every day with life. Trying to say, *I'm actually okay, I'm actually more than okay*. The information and knowledge that I have is helpful. I have much more insight and I'm lucky in the sense that it's my experiences that have given me that. So my psychiatric disability is one of the main things that has contributed to who I am today.

It is a blessing. But most people wouldn't see that. Every day in the newspaper, people are saying, *Oh, you know, you nutcase*, sort of thing. But it's given me insight, wisdom, self-awareness.

Postscript

The recovery process is more complicated than I first thought. I kept thinking, *If I can just do this, if I can just do that*. But it's not like that. It's ongoing. Even now I still have to continue looking for my real self. But I don't have any regrets. It is all worthwhile what I am doing – I am so different, so much *more*.

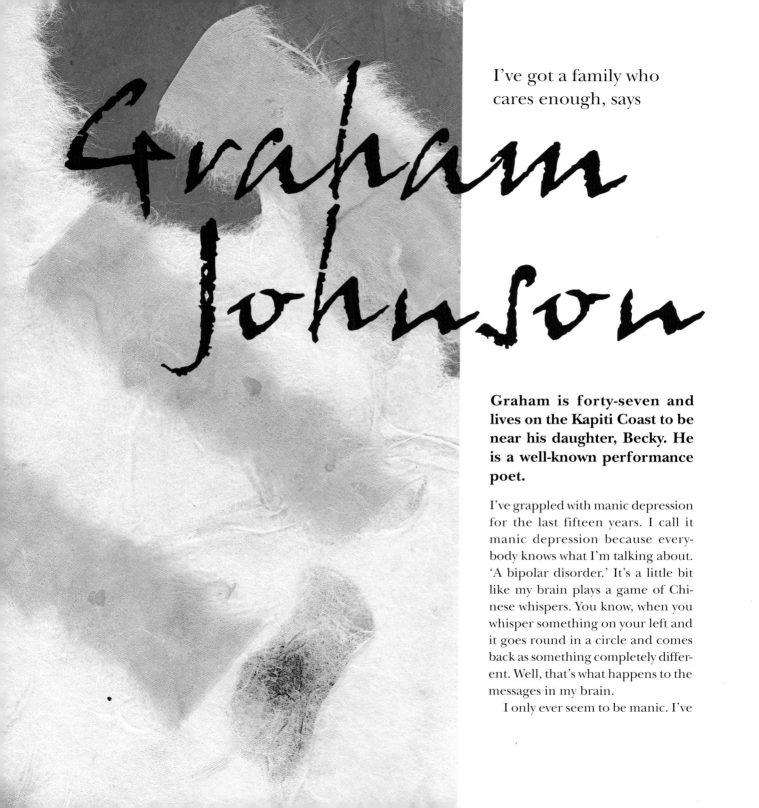

I've got a family who
cares enough, says

Graham
Johnson

**Graham is forty-seven and
lives on the Kapiti Coast to be
near his daughter, Becky. He
is a well-known performance
poet.**

I've grappled with manic depression
for the last fifteen years. I call it
manic depression because everybody knows what I'm talking about.
'A bipolar disorder.' It's a little bit
like my brain plays a game of Chinese whispers. You know, when you
whisper something on your left and
it goes round in a circle and comes
back as something completely different. Well, that's what happens to the
messages in my brain.

   I only ever seem to be manic. I've

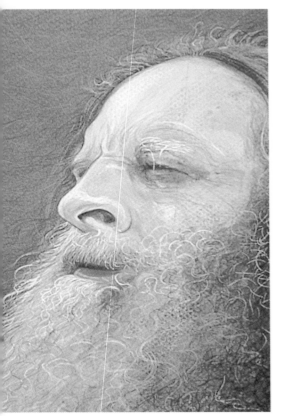

Portrait of me by Lian Hathaway, 1994.

been depressed once. I know that if I don't take medication for it, it eventually gets out of control and society can't handle me and I can't handle society. So if I want to stay having a relationship with my daughter (that's the main person, but with anybody) then I have to be medicated.

I was living in Wellink supported housing for seven years, and for six-and-a-half of them I thought I would never leave.[1] It was in an ordinary house and it was basically an ordinary flatting situation. The people I lived with were all functioning at a high level of independence. All of us needed some help in some areas, and it was all in different areas. One chap needed help with motivation. One was almost hyperactive. I really just needed that grounding under me.

We operated like a flat. We took turns at the cooking. We took turns at the shopping. We were taught to do good comparison shopping and, if we needed, there was someone to go shopping with us. Otherwise, they'd drop us off and pick us up afterwards. They came every day. When I first moved there, a support worker was living in with us. But it quickly became apparent that we were so well that this wasn't necessary.

One of the things that I liked about supported housing was that some of the needs that I'm not very good at taking care of were taken care of for me. My money. I was given my money after my expenses were taken out. So my rent was gone, my electricity bill was gone, and all I had to worry about was my food and my personal expenses. It was a real security thing. Now I'm away from that and it was a bit scary at first, but it's going well.

Now, I'm living with a couple, in their home. I've known the man for ten years, and he's one of the friends who has stood by me and been able to deal with me when I've been really unwell, really manic, and not fit to be around. Over the years my episodes have cost me a lot of friendships. People who just couldn't stand it any more and couldn't stand to have me around, even when I become well again. The memory of it is too painful. They still can't have me around and it's a real shame. That is one of the reasons I guess I make an effort to stay well.

I originally moved here from supported housing so I could be close to my girlfriend. Although that relationship hasn't worked out, I'm really glad I took that step. I didn't realise I had any independence to regain, but I suddenly feel like a free person making my own decisions surrounded by all my own things and it's just brilliant. And *that* was before I got the car!

It's really neat living here. Everything that surrounds me is mine, whereas in supported housing everything is supplied, right from soap to dish-washing liquid, to bed and dressing table. I'm like one of the family here. I'm just included and I'm made to feel welcome. Not just made to feel welcome – I'm made to feel like I belong here, and that is a wonderful thing.

I first became aware of my illness in 1984. I've always been quite impetuous, inclined to take the high road in life. But in 1984 all the clinical symptoms of bipolar disorder were there. I was thirty-two, I had a number of major stresses in my life. My father had recently died and I was still dealing with that. I'd been made redundant from my thousand-dollar-a-week job. My relationship was showing signs of cracking because of some of these other things, and on top of that I added a large bag of magic mushrooms. The outcome was a month of mayhem. People didn't know what was going on.

I mention the mushrooms because it was quite central to what happened. I took the bag and I put them in the freezer. Froze them solid, and every morning after my wife went to work I would take the bag out of the freezer, cut a slice off, and have some. I did this every day, every time I was alone in the kitchen, for the next month. I was just so far removed from reality it was hard to tell what was psychedelia and what was illness. It all became tangled up together, and it took a month before people could trick me into the hospital long enough to have somebody examine me and realise I wasn't well.

That was my first experience with manic depression and I didn't even really know what was going on at the time. I just thought I had overdone it on the mushrooms. I've smoked marijuana for over twenty-five years and for all the bad things about it (and there are lots of bad things about it) I feel that it has done me a lot of good. Before I smoked marijuana I was headed into a life of violence and possibly crime. Since then I have always taken the peaceful path.

Marijuana tends to make you look at a more peaceful way of existing and doing things. So I feel that it has been good for me in that respect and I don't think that it has contributed to a large extent to the state of my mental health. Now I find that marijuana is the only thing that cuts through the medication that I'm on and allows me to feel anything, even remotely. Marijuana helps soften that wall around my emotions, and allows a little bit to get through. I know that sounds like it's a crutch, but *I want to be able to feel things*. I don't want to spend the rest of my life a mental zombie.

The medication I take suppresses my illness or keeps it under control but it also suppresses the creativity and I really feel that the two are entwined together. So when I'm on medication I write very little. Occasionally something pushes through that fog and gets to me, and I'll write a poem, like 'Illusion'.

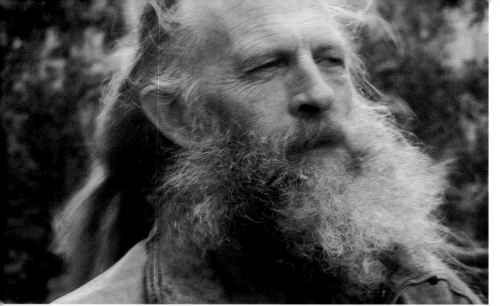

Photograph by Julie Leibrich

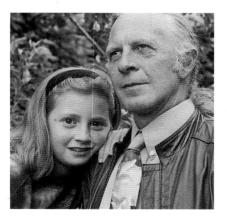

With Becky.

The first poem I wrote (on my daughter's third birthday) started an outpouring of poetry that has only been slowed down by the medication I take. But it's still there and occasionally bits come out. I've written a lot of poetry in the last ten years.[2]

I've been in and out of hospital about five times. When I first came out of hospital they gave me a large – a really large – bottle of lithium and said, *You'll have to take four of these every day for the rest of your life. Goodbye.* And so I did that for two years.

I'd shifted up to Northland, I was living out at Whangarei Heads and everyone was going swimming and boating, and I was going: *No, I think I'll go and lie on the bed and snooze or read a book.* I had no follow-up care. For two years I wasn't getting my blood tested and I had the shakes, and I was going to the toilet all the time, and I knew that it was the lithium doing this so I slowly cut it out. I was really well and healthy for another year and a half after that because I had no real stresses in my life at the time.

Then my wife became pregnant and my hours of work were cut down and things got a little tight. Then the stress seemed to spin me out and I became unwell again and I wouldn't admit it. In the end it caused the break-up of my marriage because I just accused everybody else of being sick, not me, and there was no way I was going to see a doctor. I didn't want to go back into a psychiatric hospital. So I was doing things in desperation.

I have really bright ideas when I'm unwell. They start off as bright ideas and they end up as 'I'm-grander-than-God' schemes. I came up with an idea for a training scheme to teach graphic art on computers to unemployed kids in isolated areas. It was a good scheme. The Labour Department liked it, apart from one or two points which I couldn't satisfy, so I went to some of my old friends in the gangs for the money needed.

But some of the boys were suspicious of my motives and I was given LSD (because it's hard to lie when you are on LSD). So I spent several hours, the only person who didn't have a gang patch, hallucinating and scared. In the end I was beaten up and thrown out of a truck on the side of the motorway. I was hitching to hospital when a police car stopped and picked me up. They didn't want to know. The didn't even take me to the hospital. I think I'd been raving at them from the back seat of the car and they just threw me out of their car as well. So I thought, *I'm doing well tonight. I've been thrown out by the gang* and *the police!*

It took me two days to hitchhike home. When I got there my wife had left, so I had a three-bedroom house full of gear which I gave away. Over the next few days I called people round. *You need a bookcase, don't you? Have a bookcase. You need a bedroom suite, do you? Have that.*

Then I came down to Wellington, stole my car back from my wife and lived in my car for the next three months. Because I didn't have to deal with people, I was able to be as crazy as I liked and nobody was there to tell me not to be. And all of this time I was pretty manic and then I came off that manic phase back to a level where I could see what I'd done, what I'd wrecked. And I was 500 miles away from my daughter, who meant more to me than anything.

I sat down and I wrote a poem for her third birthday, although she wasn't there. I sent it off with a nicely reasoned letter saying I'm sorry I haven't been able to be there and here's this poem for your birthday. I thought, *Now I'm well and healthy I'll get back down to Paraparaumu, and see my daughter* not realising that in the three weeks it would take me to pack up my things, get the car fixed and get to Wellington, I would move into the depression phase. Because I'd never struck that before. Nobody had ever really talked to me about it.

By the time I got to Wellington I felt so worthless that I couldn't pick up the phone and ring my ex-wife and talk to my daughter who I hadn't seen for a year, because I had nothing to offer. Every time I went to pick up the phone, I felt just a little more down and a little more useless, until in the end I decided that I had better get a job and have something to show for myself when I rang up.

I went for a job with one of the major banks as a computer operator. Got to their second level of interviews but as I walked out to the car – all neatly dressed up, the collar and tie, to go and have this interview – it struck me like a weight on my head. I couldn't go through with it. I didn't have the ability to show that I had what they needed. So I shut the roller-door in the garage, turned the car on, turned the car radio to the National Programme, which had rather nice music, and went to sleep.

I woke up in hospital. It took me three or four minutes to realise where I was and it hit me like an explosion in the head. I looked around me and just went, *Oh fuck.* My flatmate had come home unexpectedly in the after-

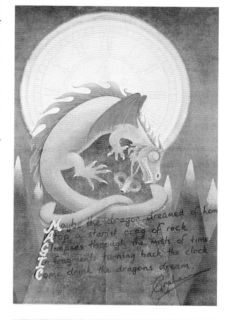

Maybe the dragon dreamed of hom...
...of a starlit crag of rock
...glimpses through the mists of time
...fragments turning back the clock
Come drink the dragons dream.

Cover of my book **Brainbows**.

noon and heard the car running in the garage and found me unconscious.

That put me in Porirua Hospital with the depression side of manic depression, and I was there for months. I can remember them saying that I had a choice between long-term villa care or ECT – shock treatment.[3] That was pretty scary. I knew that it scrambled your brain a bit. I knew that it made you lose your memory, and my one fear was that I would forget my daughter.

I had a really good doctor, Alison Brown, who was able to get my confidence and assure me that it was only transient memories that I would lose. I wouldn't lose deep-seated memories like the memory of my daughter or my family or major events in my life. So I agreed to have shock treatment. I was prescribed six shocks – and it was quite a shock, the fact that you get prescribed a shock!

I had not seen a good thing in life or around me for months and months and months at that stage. But after the third shock, I woke up the next morning, looked out the window and went, *What a nice day. What am I doing thinking what a nice day? I don't think things like that, eh?* It just did it like that, and within three weeks I was out of hospital. It was really quite amazing.

I was also lucky enough to have a key worker at that time, Bronwyn Poad who took me through the process of a really hard time with my ex-wife gaining custody of my daughter, and me having to go to the family court. She was the main reason for me being able to form a workable relationship with my ex-wife.

I've also learnt to listen to some of the professionals who I always thought were working against me. Now I've come to realise that the ones I deal with really do have my best interests at heart.

I've got a good psychiatrist, Dr Pereira, who has known me for years. It's quite hard to say what makes him good for me. He's a very tough little man – or he seems to be a very tough little man – and quite hard-line. He was quite hard-line with me for quite a long time and he was very critical of my marijuana-smoking habits. Until the day I walked into his office and he sat me down and looked at me and said, sternly, *Well, Graham, how's the marijuana smoking going?* and I went, *Really well, thank you, Doctor.* You should have seen the look on his face!

Daisy Chains

I'd rather chain daisies than people.
I'd rather sing songs than shout war.
I'd rather make friends than make money.
I'd rather have less than want more.

No cushion of wealth to surround me.
Just cushions of fern leaves and grass.
No trappings of power to confound me.
Just rainbows and love and the heavens above
To comfort as life travels past.

Graham Johnson 11/4/92.

Wild Songs – to Becky

When Daddy's sick – he must take care
And do things at his pace
And though he's sad he isn't there
He's going to win his race

When dreamers dream their wildest songs
And energy surrounds
When drummers gather all night long
And fill the night with sound.
Beware – take care
But brave the night
Let laughter be your guide
Step out and dare
To show your light
And I'll shine by your side.

Graham Johnson, 10/11/94

About four years ago, I came to a realisation. I'd often tried to meddle with my medication and my way of meddling was to get it all out of my system and then start with one pill and work up from there. It doesn't work and has put me back in hospital again, always to my surprise. Usually, it's been a conscious decision to stop my medication. *I don't care, they have to catch me first.* But this time, the last time I ended up in hospital, was a mistake.

Since then I have tried to get my medication to a point where I feel I can live with it, and I've worked out that I have to consult with the doctor. I'm happy to listen to his criticisms of what I want to do. I've ended up on less medication now than I have been on for years. There's a real two-way thing with my doctor. I actually feel that I've got some control over it and that's made all the difference. I know in myself that if I knock off the pills completely, I'll end up back in hospital. Because I did the negotiations, I can live with it. I'm happy with it, and so now I take my pills every day.

Eventually, I became a part of my family again. My ex-wife and I are friends now and it began because we both wanted to make an effort for Becky, for my daughter. My mother, too, has struggled with only some understanding of what happens to me, and has supported me in any way possible, no matter what the condition of my health. I think that is the key thing. I've got a family. I've got a family who cares enough.

Nobody puts me down. Here's an example. I was asked to go and address a school in the Hutt Valley about mental illness. It was for teachers and some of the board of trustees. I went with the Schizophrenia Fellowship Education Officer and a couple of people from Wellink. I'd done a page and a half of prose and two poems that I stood and read.

Everything went quite seemingly well. I've got the ability to read things with a bit of humour and I didn't just read it straight off, I gave them a little anecdote here and there. Then right at the end of the meeting one of the more antagonistic parents piped up and said, *And how should we tell our children to behave if they meet one of* your *people on the street?* There was dead silence. I leaned forward and said, *Politely.*

It was a really good note to end the meeting on. It sounds really funny, but it's really true – the best thing you can treat anybody with is politeness and chances are they'll respond in kind. It doesn't matter if they're ill or not. I guess that's how I deal with almost everything in life, with gentleness, politeness and respect, and I guess that's why I get those things back.

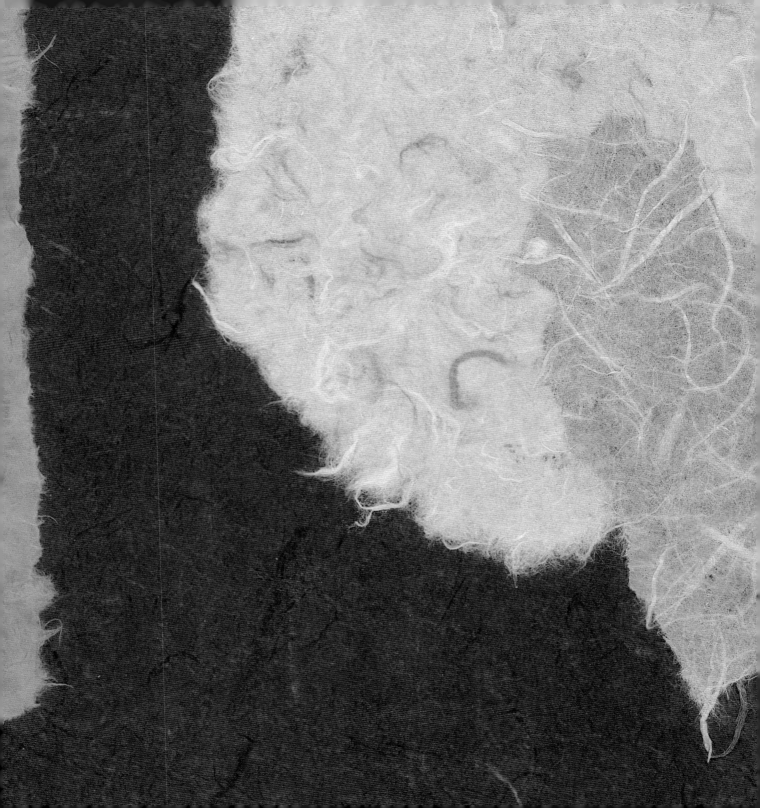

It's playtime now, says

Pat Cumming

Pat is forty-eight and works on the Kapiti Coast as manager of a large community centre. She is also a Justice of the Peace.

I suffered from depression most of my life, which was bouts of total blackness. I couldn't get out of bed, just wanted to stick my head under the pillow, and I had some slight feelings that I wanted to do myself in. This began in my late teens. And during my twenties I had bouts of what people call 'burning out'.

I've managed to work and keep myself going over those years, and just learnt to live with it. I've been to various doctors and some have given me antidepressants, which I hated, because they made my hands tingle, and I felt like a zombie. I've been told that I just needed to raise my self-esteem and learn how to confront people and just be a bit more assertive. So I did all of those sorts of things, but nothing changed.

Over the last ten years I have made incredible leaps forward in my own personal growth. But it was still there. Funny that.

So about four years ago I talked to yet another doctor, a *new* doctor, and he said had I ever considered that I might have a chemical imbalance? And I said, *Well, no, I hadn't.* No one had ever talked to me about that. I was an addictions counsellor, and even though I knew something about chemical imbalance, I thought that people with depression felt powerless about something in their lives and just needed to make some life changes.

The doctor suggested that I go onto a medication called aropax. He wanted me to go away and think about it, but I wasn't very willing. Mostly because I felt ashamed of the fact that I had a mental illness and was a counsellor and so should be able to deal with it. That good guilt word *should*! I *should* be able to deal with it – like pull my socks up and get on with it.

I had worked in a mental health field, you see, as a support worker with people with mental illness. I was a trained addiction counsellor, and a lot of people looked up to me and asked me for guidance. And here I was – seemingly, I couldn't even handle my own life. It was huge. It was like *physician heal thyself.* I mean, it's just not on really. You've got to be the one that's on top of things. But it's a myth – like there are many myths in our lives. I don't believe that one any more.

Things were good in my life, my relationship was going well, my work was going well, I had everything to be thankful for, but I always had this *little dark cloud* that sat over my shoulder. It just hovered above my shoulder. It followed me round and took something away from me. I'd never been so debilitated that I couldn't work. I'd functioned, but there would be mornings when I would get up and just feel low within myself for no particular reason.

So I talked to my closest friend and gave it a lot of thought. In the end I decided to give it a go, because the doctor *did* assure me that if I didn't have a chemical imbalance, it wouldn't work.

Well it worked! It took about a week or so but it was like

My Home

This is the place that I love the best,
A little brown house, like a ground-bird's nest,
Hid among grasses, and vines and trees,
Summer retreat of the birds and the bees.

The tenderest light that ever was seen
Sifts through the vine-made window screen–
Sifts and quivers, and flits and falls
On home-made carpets and grey-hung walls.

All through June, the west wind free
The breath of the clover brings to me.
All through the languid July day
I catch the scent of the new-mown hay.

The morning glories and scarlet vine
Over the doorway twist and twine;
And every day, when the house is still,
The humming-bird comes to the window-sill.

In the cunningest chamber under the sun
I sink to sleep when the day is done;
And am waked at morn, in my snow-white bed,
By a singing-bird on the roof o'erhead.

Ella Wheeler Wilcox

coming out of the dark. It was like coming out of a tunnel into the sunshine. The difference in me was incredible. Where I used to drag myself up the driveway at the end of the day, I had a spring in my step again, and I actually coped a lot better with any stress that came along. I was a lot calmer and quite a bit nicer to be with, more positive.

I've been on the tablets for two years, and, to start off with, found life a lot better. But more recently I've seen my health go downhill, a gradual thing where finally this year I've felt exhausted and, at times, I've had that feeling of depression coming back. I could be driving to work and a little voice will say, *Why don't you just drive off the road and get it over and done with?* Or just not wanting to get up, wanting to sleep forever. Not being able to cope with things.

So I started to look into a more natural way of trying to deal with this. I have been going to a natural health practitioner – she's particularly sensible and has been a nurse. So there's none of this *Well, we're just going to chuck that out the window, you won't need that any more.* We hope that I can go off the medication at some stage, as I don't want to be on it for the rest of my life.

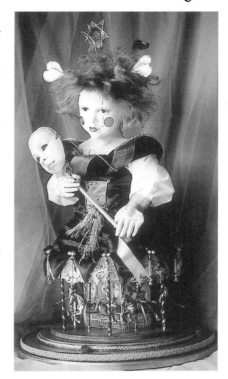

Paradox

I would never say to anyone *don't take your medication,* because there are some people I know who do function a lot better and their life is enhanced by it. And I see the difference that medication made for me initially.

Even though I could see that, because I was ashamed, I held back from telling people, but I have no problem with that now. I believe that my experiences have enhanced my life and given me an understanding of mental illness. So now I can relate to people with mental illness in a more positive way, with understanding and empathy, rather than fear.

My mum was hard to tell because she's from the 'old school' and she has the old idea of mental illness. Just helping her to understand that I was okay, and what I was doing, was a good thing for me. But, yes, it was hard to tell her because of that stigma in her head about people with mental illness.

I do have a mental illness. It took a while to accept that, but I certainly wouldn't be on aropax if I didn't, because it is a medication for people who have mental illness.

I didn't really think much about having a mental illness until I had to go to the Mental Health Team for counselling when my mother was ill and I needed someone to talk to. Then I realised that on my file there, and at my doctor's, was this thing that said I suffer from depression. It would be classed as a mental illness and I was in the system. And it's already gone against me with life insurance. When I applied for life insurance, I was honest when I filled the form out. Then another form was sent to my doctor to document

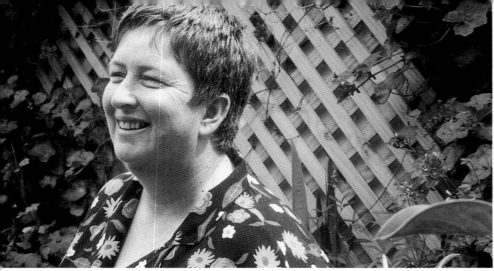

Photograph by Julie Leibrich

my history of depression. And my premium costs me more than other people's – all for being honest, all for suffering from depression.

I'm a great believer in the Serenity Prayer.[1] I'm not a Christian, but I believe there are some things I have to accept that I can't change, and I can certainly help myself. Recently, for instance, I've been getting in touch with my inner child.

When I was about thirteen I was sexually abused by a friend's husband, and carried that knowledge, without sharing it with anybody, for about twenty-five years. I couldn't talk about it and I carried this burden, this guilt, this shame. I have a feeling that's where my depression came from.

I believe that in all of us there is a child that is with us from day one. And that there are very many parts of that child. The one I have focused on is the wounded child. I needed to do some work on my own wounded inner child, and I needed to help her to work through the abuse and grow up and be able to deal with things differently.

The inner child is the essence that is you. It makes you the person that you are. It's a part of you that hides deep inside of you, particularly if you have been abused – whatever kind of abuse – and a lot of the scars are on the inside.

It's the *real* you, who knows the truth about things, who knows you, and knows what you're capable of. You're born with that essence. As you grow up, your public figure becomes very distorted. You learn ways to cope, you learn ways to get your own way, but your inner child pops up every now and again – like when you stamp your foot, or sometimes when you're sick and, you know, you just want your mum. That's really the only time that a lot of people are actually aware that there is a child inside.

About seven years ago, I started talking to my inner child and asked her what her name was. She said, *Patrice.* I started listening to Patrice and she was very hurt about the sexual abuse and very scared of men. Over the years (when I didn't even know her name) she used to try and tell me how she felt. But I pushed her deeper inside and said, *I don't want anything to do with you. You're scary. You've got all the memories. You remember all that stuff and I don't want to remember that as an adult, thank you very much. So you can just go down there somewhere and be quiet.* So I treated her like my parents treated me. In other words, I ignored her.

For the last eight years, I've been helping Patrice, the essence that is me, to come out. Off and on I did intensive healing work, on my own, and sometimes with the help of people who had the skills to help me.

For the last couple of years Patrice and I have played. It's playtime now. We've *done* all that stuff, we know each other and I love her very much. I think she's very special, and so we play and we do lots of drawing, and lots of writing.

Patrice has this Indian head-dress that she wears with lots of brightly coloured feathers, so I wear that sometimes with friends. I've dragged everybody else in on this, you see! I've got a friend called Tottie, and a friend called Jennifer Jane, and I've got a friend called Sydney, a girl. And my sister's Poppy, and I've got Annie, Rosebud, and Jasmine. So I've got seven friends and every now and again, we get together and we have an inner child party and we do our drawing. Oh, we think it's really cool! And sometimes we even make bubbles!

Sometimes if I have a really good day, I come home and I get my art set out (a $9.99 art set from The Warehouse, which has 100 felts and 50 pencils and a rubber!). Patrice thinks that's wonderful because she was never allowed one of those when she was a kid. I'll draw her in the car with her hair flying out the window and everybody happy.

So it's helped me incredibly to get to know Patrice, and she's absolutely marvellous, she's so much fun. She's such a strong little girl, eh? And so brave. She likes Cowboys and Indians. She's got a big silver sheriff's badge that she wears. One time Sydney and Tottie and Patrice went to Levin to see *Batman and Robin.* And we all went to the Toy Warehouse beforehand, and I bought the Indian head-dress and the sheriff's badge.

The inner child work has made me more of a whole person

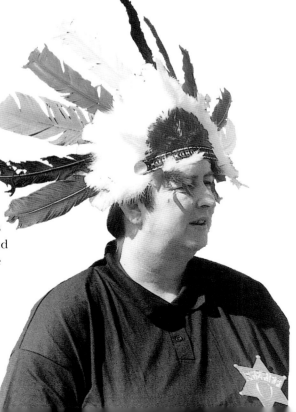

Patrice in her favourite gear.

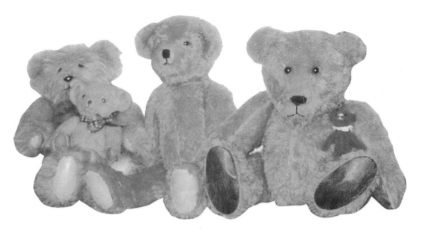

Friends for life.

and made me love and appreciate who I am. The *whole* me.

Now, if I felt that I wasn't having a good day I would be less inclined to stick my head under the pillow. I have more strategies. I believe that finding someone and talking to them is helpful, and being open about what's wrong with me rather than trying to hide it. I think the shame and the guilt stuff is really crippling because that's the stuff that puts you to bed and puts your head under the pillow and you don't want to see anybody.

Now I can say, *Look, I'm not feeling so good today. Can I come and talk to you* or *Can I just come and be with you?* I would never have been able to do that years ago. I can remember sitting in the bath sobbing, and I had a flatmate who was very, very good to me and I didn't speak to her for a week. I just completely withdrew. But I don't see it as a good way for me any more. I know it's hard sometimes not to withdraw, but I've got to actually make the effort to talk.

I've got good friends. And I've got a dog. I just love having him around because you've got to do something. You've got to look after him – I mean he can't get his dog roll out of the fridge! He's always a good excuse to go for a walk, too.

I'm a great gatherer, especially in the winter. I like going out on a cold winter's day. I like getting into nature and I like gathering bird's nests and leaves and stones. I also love photography and I sometimes photograph nature's patterns. I really like being able to get out in the fresh air with someone that I'm very comfortable with, who likes gathering as well. And just, you know, spending a nice day. Hop in the car, head north, no further than Levin probably. Have a nice lunch somewhere, cup of coffee, and then do the gathering and just come back at night feeling really tired but happy with all these treasures, lichen and bird's nests and stones.

It's a whole thing, it's a lifestyle, it may be medication, it may be having to have a rest in the afternoon, eating a certain way, things like that. It's making sure I get enough sleep and do healthy things. Balance. There's the physical and the mental, and then there's the spiritual side which I think people forget completely. It's really important for me to get in touch with my spiritual side as well.

I have my own spiritual beliefs which are very basic. I believe there is a power greater than me. It's based on the twelve-step program of AA, that a power greater than me can restore me to sanity. Being in touch with my higher power is very important to me. I don't consciously connect with my higher power every day, but I know that my higher power is there, that's the strange thing. If you're not too rigid about it, it does actually become part of you.

Part of one of the steps is *When you are wrong, promptly admit it.* I try and follow that philosophy as much as I can, like making amends with people, not letting things go on and on. Being honest with people about where I'm at and how I feel about them. If someone hurts me, being able to go and say to them, *I feel really hurt.* It takes a lot of the stress of life away.

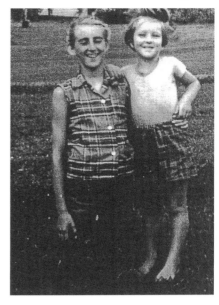

Patrice and her big sister.

I just stay in the day. I used to be a great scriptwriter, you know, about what was going to happen out there, and who was going to say what, and how things were going to turn out. I'd destroy any enjoyment before I had actually got there. Instead of stressing and straining and getting angry and uptight because things aren't going the way that I want, I try and go with the flow more and just accept that's how it is.

I think spirituality is the one thing that is lacking a lot with people – but it's got to be their *own* spirituality. Belief in a higher power has helped me to understand that whatever happens to me in my life is meant to be. I'm here today for a reason. I don't know why, it could be for someone else, it could be for me. It could be for you.

Postscript

I came off medication in April 1998. My mother died the following June and I got through the grief process without needing to go back on the medication. I just practised my philosophy of allowing myself to feel, talk to people, and listen to Patrice. My spiritual beliefs also gave me a lot of strength.

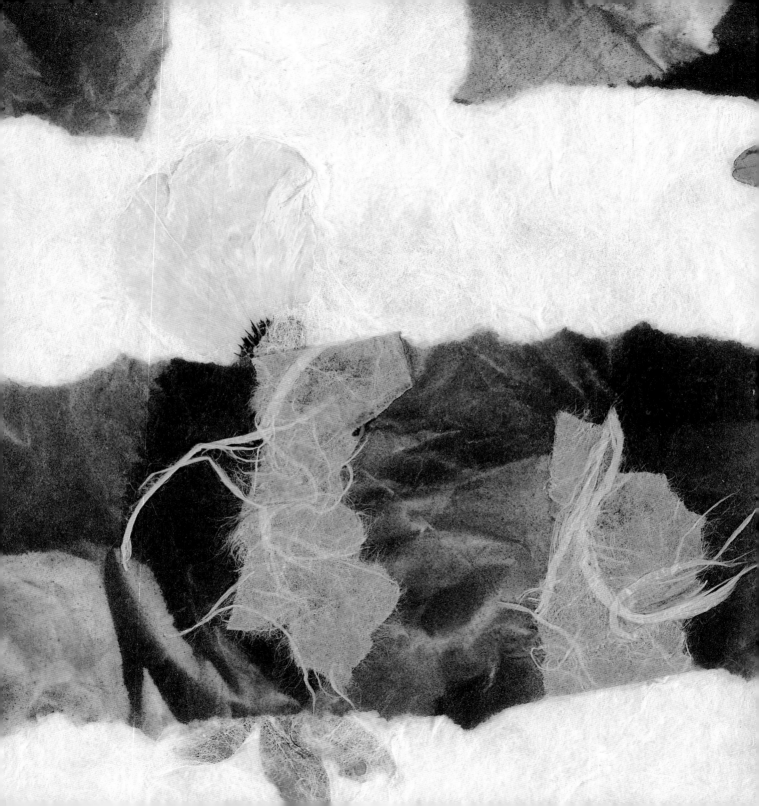

It's all about managing my life, says

Susan Butler

Susan is forty-four and lives in Dunedin. She is a trained typist/receptionist. She loves her cats and her garden.

Anxiety is like when you sit an exam or fly in an aeroplane. You get anxious – but where this is taken to the extreme, you can't move. And it's constant. It's always there. It doesn't matter what you think, anxiety is like the seed of doubt, so you're always doubting.

When I was thirteen, I was hospitalised for six months because in those days that's what they did. I was taken away from my family and put in a hospital. I was mis-diagnosed as schizophrenic and I had all kinds of drugs tried out on me. It's very hard for me now to take any form of medication, which in some ways works against me becoming well.

I became unwell again at seventeen, at twenty-one, at twenty-six, and thirty-four. It was when I became unwell at twenty-six that I was finally told I had an anxiety disorder. All this time, because of the way it was in the mental health scene, I was unaware of what was wrong with me. I was told it was a behavioural problem, so I looked upon myself as weak and I punished myself, and I did that right up until I was thirty-six years of age. And that is just so wrong.

All of the times that I've been ill have been set off by very big stresses in my life. When I was thirteen it was set off when I went to high school, because I had been over-protected as a child. I just couldn't cope with becoming independent, so that was a major stress.

When I was seventeen I feel that it was because of my relationship with my father. My father was English and behind glass. He was very affectionate to me until I was seven, and then because of the way that men relate to women he felt that it was improper to be affectionate. I probably felt that I'd done something wrong, that he had withdrawn that affection. He was very affectionate until I was about seven, and then he had to be proper.

I actually had a very good relationship with my father. Now when I look back (my father passed away last year) he was a very, very forward-looking man in women's issues. When I was eighteen, my father had a talk to me when he was digging the garden. *Do not feel you have to become married*, he said. *You do everything that you feel is important for you and you get married when you feel like it*. Knocked my socks off! We had also had several discussions over the years where he believed that women should not be treated as incubators. Very, very forward-thinking man.

About five years ago, I had to ask him, *Do you love me?* Because that was a very important issue for me. It's very funny because it's true what they say about the stages of life. It was just before I was forty and I was going through my mid-life crisis. There were issues that I had to deal with and that was one of them. He answered, *Of course I do*, behind a book or something.

My father could not understand anxiety. He could not understand depression. He had great difficulty dealing with it. He left everything to my mother to deal with, which was sad because I needed the support of both my parents. He never visited me until after my mum died when I was twenty-one, which was very difficult for me.

But I understand their difficulties now, because then there was not much information around. They didn't know what was happening to me. And I feel very sorry for my mother – she died before I actually knew about my illness. In fact I said to my father, *When you pass away, and if you meet Mum, please tell her that I had anxiety, that it wasn't her fault.* Because I can remember when I was seventeen she took me to hospital and she went away crying. That was very hard for me, very very hard for me, because I think she felt that she'd failed as a mother. And she hadn't at all. If anything, she'd done too much.

I was over-protected as a child. I felt that I couldn't cope because my mother had made all these decisions for me. I had, in effect, become tied to my mother. Therefore I didn't grow and didn't cope as an individual by myself. Then I went into this relationship with my husband. But because of my background, I hadn't grown and couldn't cope as a person by myself emotionally. Do you understand that?

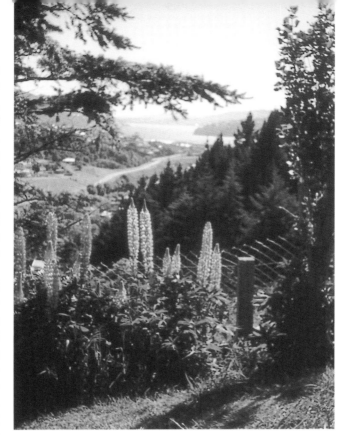

View from my garden.

So there he was. My safe person that I needed in order to cope. But he treated me very badly. He eroded my confidence, everything about me. To a point where I was a shell. And when he left I got very ill. I was quite unrealistic about my husband. I saw him through rose-coloured glasses. I mean, I really loved him. But he abused that. He used that against me.

My marriage broke down when I was thirty-four, and I went with it. I have been sick since then – for ten years. It's the worst I have ever been in my whole life. Before that I used to be sick for a year, eighteen months at the most, and then I'd live a normal life until I got ill again, but this time it's been different. It's just devastated me, devastated, total devastation. But going through this illness, for me, has been an acceptance, and a growing process, and a learning to like myself as I am.

It's taken all this time to build myself up again and become whole and actually feel good about myself as a person. To be able to stand alone as a person. It's been a very, very long process. It's taken me years to be able to deal with it. I've had to develop my own strategies as to how to cope. It's all about managing my life and doing things for myself that don't bring on anxiety.

Now they've done more research, and I've bought a very good book about anxiety and phobias.[1] I haven't got phobias, but anxiety. I realise there is a combination of factors that contribute. There are environmental factors, there are chemical imbalances, and of course there are behaviours that are learnt when you are growing up. So it is actually a combination and I have stopped bashing myself and finally accepted that I am not a weak person.

Anxiety is very crippling. I lose my independence and I can't go anywhere at all without having somebody with me. It has altered my life so dramatically. I wanted to be a kindergarten teacher: I couldn't. I wanted to have children, and I made the choice not to. My whole life just goes on hold because I can't do anything because I'm so anxious. My home is my safe place. It's been a real struggle for me even to go out and feel comfortable. I can drive so far, but then I might have a panic attack. It's a very hard thing to actually put into words.

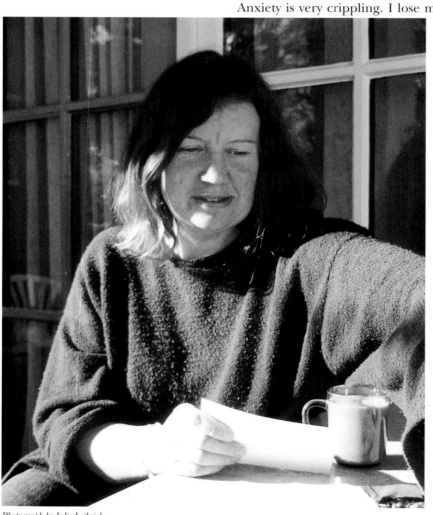

Panic attacks are very different for different people. With me, I get very, very hot and I feel like something really bad is going to happen to me. Reassurance and all those things go out the window, and your bodily symptoms totally engulf you.

With anxiety you hyperventilate. I found the best way to deal with that is to suck a lolly – sucking it regulates my breathing, and it also wets my mouth. (This may sound ridiculous), I feel that the sucking action is a comfort.

With panic attacks I find the best

Photograph by Julie Leibrich

thing (oh, sometimes I just don't cope), is to go to my neighbour's. She's very good. She'll come over, sit on the end of the bed, and we just have a yap about other things. I can't focus on what's happening to me – we have to talk and then I'm fine. I get up and I get a cold face-cloth and I find if I cool myself down, talk to myself a bit, read a book, the adrenalin rush and all the other things associated with it will slowly go down.

I used to have the attacks during the day, but I don't now. I wake up into a panic attack which is terrifying, because I have no idea what the stimulus is. If you've got no idea what starts it, how can you deal with it? I've got no idea, so I go to the bathroom and cool myself down and I talk to myself. *Go away*. I have to do this. *Just go away! I'm all right. No, I'm not poisoned by the fish I ate*. And I'll read.

Sometimes I just have to go to hospital and they put me on medication, which is a really big issue for me. I'm scared I'm going to get side-effects because I seem to be drug sensitive. And I stay there. The other issue with anxiety is that safety is of the utmost importance. It's a very, very subtle thing, I become institutionalised almost immediately. I mean I'm quite an intelligent person, but it's so subtle that I'm not even aware that it's happening.

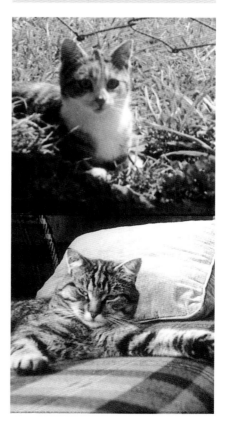

Moozie (top), and Tiger.

I feel safe, I want to stay in this nice little area, so we have to get onto the medication. We have to shove it down my throat and I've got to be very brave and pace up and down and wait for twenty minutes to see if I'm going to have any side-effects. And that issue for me, in itself, raises extra levels of anxiety.

I've had so many different medications. I'm very lucky, I'm on a new medication now that has no side-effects, absolutely marvellous, no dry mouth. I'm on aropax. I'm very, very lucky that it suits me. It doesn't suit a lot of people, but I'm very, very lucky that it suits me.

My psychiatrist suggested that I go to the Cameron Centre and have some counselling.[2] It was very, very hard for me because I had really bad anxiety and I had to drive there and drive home, after those terrible sessions. But I'm very lucky that I'm quite a strong person with a very strong survival instinct, and I made myself do it. I would not have been able to get through these past ten years if I hadn't had that strength.

Going for counselling was the best thing I ever did. I had a whole year at Presbyterian Support, and I just talked. I talked about when I was a child, my relationship with my father, about what it was like being married – I just talked and talked. I was amazed at my emotional response to some of the things I talked about. That was the best thing that I ever did. I'd recommend it to anyone. I actually faced up to all those things and dealt with them, and it was like a cleansing, really. When I dealt with all the issues I had through counselling, it was like a new phase of my life opened for me, which was absolutely marvellous.

Also, I had the steady support of Karen Harris, my district nurse. She's the most marvellous person. If I won a million dollars in Lotto, I'd give her one hundred thousand. She was always there. Nothing was ever too much for her. She was understanding. A lot of district nurses aren't like that, but … she's the pick of the bunch. My father and sister always disappeared and locked themselves in other rooms when I got ill, but Karen was always there for me.

She's been my main support since 1989. You see, before then there was nothing like that in place. It was very, very difficult. But this time, thank goodness, she was given to me as my district nurse. And she would come and visit me on a weekly basis. Then it got down to two-weekly, and we worked through all the different issues that were with me, and she's just supported me all the way.

My cats, my garden and my sister and her children. Especially her children. Her children have just done so much in building my confidence. When I've been in hospital I can't go straight home because I live by myself. So I go and stay with my sister. Then one of the children will come and stay with me at my home for the weekend, so that I can adjust. This also happens when I start to drive again. One of them will always come with me until I build up a level of confidence to drive by myself.

The major thing for me about keeping well is the support. Without my sister's children I don't know how I would have got on. My district nurse and my sister's children have been the most important thing to me.

I've got two cats and they're really lovely. It's important to have animals. The first cat I got was a stray who had been treated really badly, so she wasn't exactly loving. I got myself another kitten, which I brought up. It's really important to have something to love, and something to love me. When I have a panic attack, it's important my cat's there because he's a comfort to me. I have to live as normal a life as possible. I talk to my cats and treat them like they're people. It takes my mind off me.

I have quite a big garden, which I have created myself. That has saved me. Whenever I have felt bad, I've gone out into my garden and I'm so busy thinking of bloody weeds that it takes my focus off *me*.

Also, right from when I was very young, I made a conscious decision not to keep in contact with anybody that I met in hospital.

I live in a state house unit which I want to buy, but I haven't got much hope of that on the benefit – the invalid's benefit. My rent's $101 a week, and I get $115 a week in my hand. I've been on less than that for years. That is another demoralising aspect of being ill. Not only do you have to deal with your illness, and the side-effects of your medication, you have to deal with having no money. That's why people become angry at politicians. You get angry, and they treat you like you're nothing.

And professional people! I had a doctor once who was so patronising. I said to him I have actually got an anxiety disorder, not an intellectual disability. A lot of doctors are like that. They treat you like you're stupid. But why do professionals think that you can treat anxiety like it's a coat that you can just take off and throw away? It is not that easy. Anxiety is with me for my life. I can't take it off and throw it away. I'm very intelligent. I want myself as I am. Accept myself. I like myself now. I like my honesty, my truthfulness, the fact that I can, if people tell me things, keep a secret. The fact that I'm respectful of people. Just lots of things. It's time to do things for me, and to look after me and to love myself.

I wrote a list of things that I want to do before I die. There are lots of things, just small things. I want to learn how to ride a horse. I want to learn to play the flute. I want to get my heavy traffic licence and I want to go on the Brass Monkey Rally. [3]

On Tuesday night I did the Baldwin Street Gut Buster.[4] It was 30 degrees, and I got three-quarters of the way up. I thought I could just go back down. But my mother brought me up with proverbs, and one of them was: *If you cheat, you're only cheating yourself.* And I thought, *No! If I go back down, I'll know that I haven't done this darn walk.* So I wet my face again with my flannel, and drank a bit more water, and I got to the top!

Postscript

When I got the draft of the story I was really scared. I read a few excerpts out to my sister. Then, later in the afternoon, I read the whole thing and I felt really good. I thought, *this is how it's really been for me.*

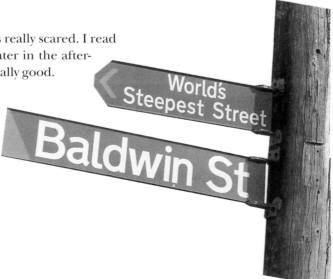

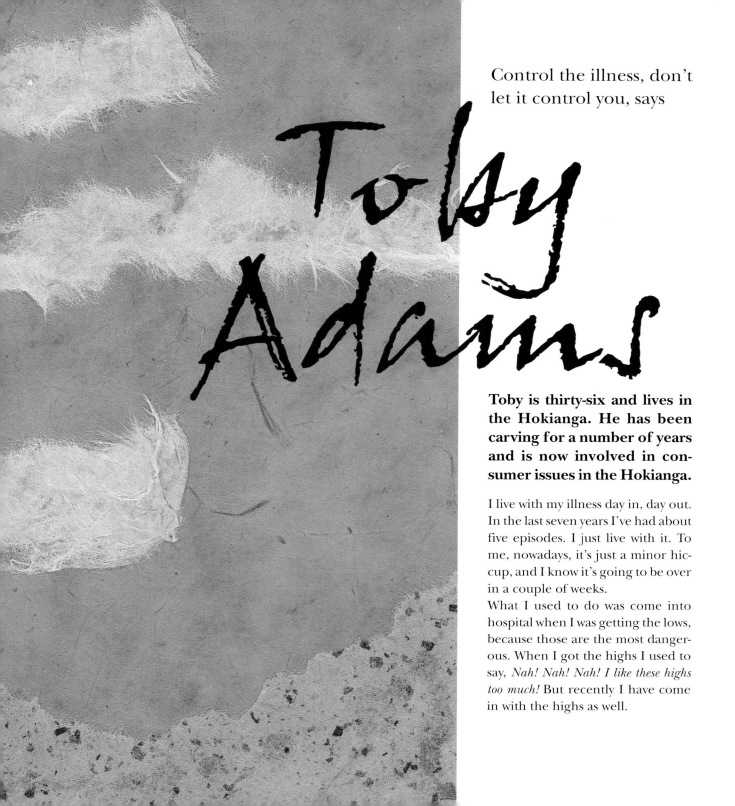

Control the illness, don't let it control you, says

Toby Adams

Toby is thirty-six and lives in the Hokianga. He has been carving for a number of years and is now involved in consumer issues in the Hokianga.

I live with my illness day in, day out. In the last seven years I've had about five episodes. I just live with it. To me, nowadays, it's just a minor hiccup, and I know it's going to be over in a couple of weeks.

What I used to do was come into hospital when I was getting the lows, because those are the most dangerous. When I got the highs I used to say, *Nah! Nah! Nah! I like these highs too much!* But recently I have come in with the highs as well.

Opposite: detail from **Child of the Sea.** This carving tells the story of Opo, the dolphin. I also wrote the poem which is carved in the top right corner of the mural:

As the river flowed the sea stirred,
   a child of the sea came.
He came into the hearts of a people
who played and swam with this child
   – a child of the sea.

I'm lucky. I'm one of the lucky ones. I've got tremendous insight. I know what's happening on the inside and I know that I'm going off the rocks. My train of thought is not normal. I'm thinking that somebody's a king or something. I've realised the thoughts I'm having are not normal. It's a slow realisation, but I *realise*.

The highs are usually also accompanied by lack of sleep. So when I haven't been sleeping for a couple of days and I've been up all night, I know something's up. But as most psychiatric people know, once you get into that world you become part of it and it's real hard to break away. When you're in the world of fantasy you become part of that world. That's the trouble with it.

My fantasy worlds are pretty good. They can be very very pleasurable. It's hard to describe what it's like to be high to someone who hasn't had the experience. It's a drug; it's a drug. It's like cocaine. It's like heroin. And I actually look stoned when I'm high. Only, we don't need to take anything to get that high.

I'm also lucky that I live in a small town where the people around me know that I'm a psychiatric patient. So when things are a bit strange they can let my nurse know, *Look, Toby's not …*

When I say I want to go to hospital, I usually go to hospital. There's not much mucking around. The last time it happened I was hospitalised for two weeks. I hadn't been in hospital for two years. And a week later I was back at work.

I've been on lithium since I was sixteen. They have experimented with other tablets in the past and they haven't worked. Now it's lithium and nulactil pericyazine.

For myself, I cannot see how you can recover from mental illness. Well, I never have. I know I'm going to have an episode in the future, and there's not much I can do about it. It's just living with it – coping with it to a level where you have a good enough existence of life.

It's not like you're a drug addict. Once an addict stops taking drugs, then they can recover, and if they keep away from the drug they do recover. That's not the case with manic depression. Manic depression will sneak up on you when you least expect it, and there is no way that it's not going to come back. It always does. It always does. It's just a matter of learning how to cope with it. When you have an episode, try and keep it compact, try and keep the damage area closed in. Control the illness, don't let the illness control you.

I'm very, very lucky at Rawene, because they understand that here and I keep these episodes as far apart as I possibly can. I used to have about eight or nine episodes a year. Now I have one every two or three years.

I have mini-episodes when I can feel something's happening and I see my nurse and say, *Look, this has happened to me*. And we change the situation where I'm living. I move out of the situation I'm in. I find somewhere else to live. I find ways of coping.

When you have a family, problems can put you under stress, and if you're under stress you're not going to sleep. If you don't sleep you're going to have an episode. It's simple as that.

Rest is important, too. Sometimes when I'm totally exhausted I will go to sleep at five o'clock in the afternoon and wake up in the morning. Yeah, I like my long sleeps. If I'm tired I usually will have something to eat and then just relax on my bed and crash out. It's easier to combat your illness when you're nice and rested than it is when you're exhausted, because if you're exhausted you're opening up the door for the adrenaline rush.

In my lifetime I've come across three good nurses. Psychiatric doctors – you only talk to them for about five minutes and that's the end of it. They don't really cope with you day to day. But nurses … The nurse that I have now would have to be the best I've ever come across. He saw something in me and decided to give me a job, and he's still trudging away at it. I have nothing but respect for the guy. Yeah!

I have friends in the town that make sure that I've got contact. I'm not really a loner, but I have learnt how to be alone. But if I want company I'll find it. The biggest problem I have is that I haven't got a vehicle. My family are only about forty ks away but it's across the river. Sometimes I hitchhike over.

Three years ago, it was brought to my attention that there was a position called community support worker up for grabs, and I was asked to apply. I had no idea what it was, but it was explained to me that it was something to do with mental health, so I thought, *Why not? I'll do it*.

I went to the interview with my father. He was my support. The interview was choice. We were sitting there and Dad gave me fantastic support. It was the first

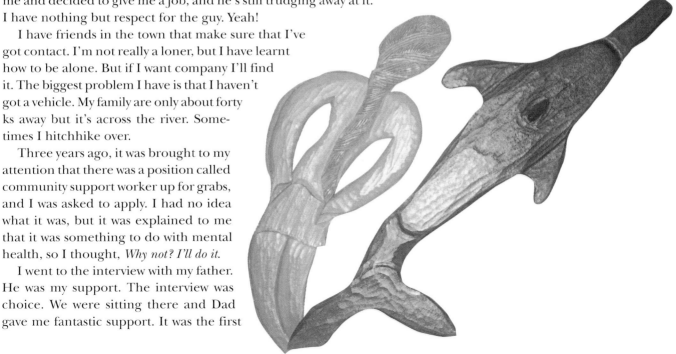

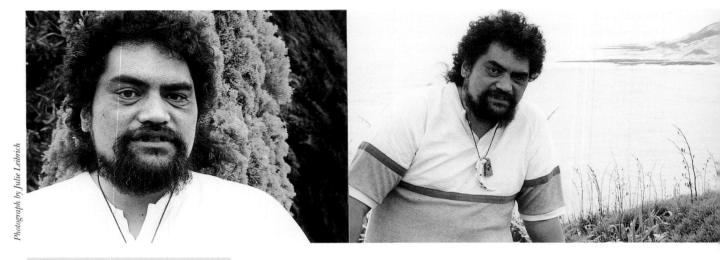

Photograph by Julie Leibrich

This is me at Arai-te-Uru.

time I'd heard my father talk about this, you know. I'd given this man a hard time most of my life, and he was saying things like, *Well, when my son finds that there's a problem, he'll find a practical solution to it.* He's saying all these things and I was going, *Wow!* It was great to hear that. Dad really was there for me. I nailed the interview halfway through.

Basically what a community support worker does is look after any social welfare problems the client has. He makes sure his living arrangements are okay, the rent is paid, or if he's staying with family, the family's okay. He makes sure he's getting his medication and that things are not getting too hard. Tries to make life easier. If the family situation is not working or the caregiver situation's not working, you try and find other accommodation. You've got a whole team to back you up. We do it that way.

I'm also the chairman of the consumer group we're trying to start up here. And it's quite good because I'm the link between the consumers and the community support worker team, and we keep it nice and tight.

Working as a mental health worker is a positive experience for me. I've been able to turn a negative into a positive. It's up to you what you do with it. To me, mental illness is just another illness. It's like being diabetic – it's just something you have to live with. The point is people are not afraid of diabetics.

The trouble is that the only exposure we have in the media is the bad things that happen (like Raurimu and Aramoana). You don't hear about the positive things people with mental illness do.

There are people who are criminally insane; there are also people that use insanity as a line of defence. But most people with a mental illness are good people – they've got families, they hold down a job, they're just trying to exist like anyone else. It's not the life I expected.

The only real negative thing I have with this illness I've got is that it stopped me having my dream. I actually wanted to be a professional wrestler. But once I went into Kingseat at sixteen that was the end of that dream.[1] There was no way I was going to be an athlete after that.

From sixteen to twenty, I was in hospital twenty times. In one way I was lucky that the illness affected me young and that I grew up with it and have learned how to cope with it. Some people never learn how to cope with it; it just takes them over every time. Me, I've learned to live with it. I think mostly because of insight. I was able to see what was happening and realise that I could make changes. I was never going to find a cure, but I was going to be able to live out the good times and ride the bad times, and that's the way my life was going to have to be.

A lot of things helped. Like carving. When I turned twenty-one, I got into carving, and it gave me confidence. I wasn't a nutter, I was somebody who could do something. I used to be a full-time carver. Carving is 70 per cent skill and 30 per cent imagination. I was taught you're a storyteller, so you're relaying a story in the carving. I never mixed up the characters that I was carving with my fantasy. Carving was always a job to me. It was a skill.

Playing sport – that helped a lot, too. Sport is another confidence thing. I used to be badly co-ordinated and being on drugs all the time slowed down my reaction time. But I've played sports like netball, basketball, rugby, golf, table tennis. They're fun, and the more fun things you can do, the more enjoyable life is. Then you also have a reason for being around.

I haven't got any kids or a wife so I've got to think of reasons why I'm still going to be here the next morning. You know, and for my own satisfaction. And helping people out is a good way to go. As for the questions about why I can cope … sometimes I can't. But I just keep on trucking on, hoping that around the corner something good's going to happen to me. And I stay around for that.

I'm learning how to be a Christian, to be honest. They talk a lot about forgiving. I've found out life's a lot happier when you don't worry about it. If you're going to move on you have to forgive. If you keep going back to the past, *He did this to me, he did that to me*, there's going to be no positive outcome.

It took me a long time to forgive my father for not letting me become a wrestler, but I realised that I wouldn't have become one anyway, not with this illness. As for being chucked into lockup rooms and tied down and given injections, those people are only doing their jobs. Something had to be done, you know, I couldn't carry on in society the way I was going. And if I hadn't ended up in hospital, I probably would have ended up in prison. So something had to be done.

I've always been interested in writing stories. At a very young age it was noticeable that I couldn't read or write. I took remedial reading and had a special tutor, which is why I can read very well, but I can't write. I've taken adult classes, but I just can't spell properly. So what I do is I write phonetically, and then translate it to someone else who then writes it down. It's hard, but that's how I do it.

As I said, I'm a carver, so I'm a storyteller. I always have stories running through my head, and with the completion of this last story I thought maybe I could get pen to paper, and write a few more. So there's always that around the corner.

The story I'm putting in this book is called 'The Room'. Remembering and revealing this was painful. At the time that it happened I was in a very high state and putting it to paper was done from the bits and pieces that I remember, some very vividly. But I felt I had to, as it is a story which should be told, for those who have been through it and for those who will go through it, and for the families of those who have been in the room.

At Opononi, beside the statue of Opo, the dolphin.

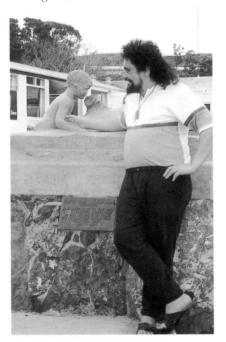

It is about a room called seclusion. It is where you are forced into when you become uncontrollable or are a danger to yourself or others. Nowadays seclusion is a controlled environment where there is a camera to make sure you are safe, and medication is on a regular basis; also you are given time to go to the toilet and, if you are a smoker, time out for a cigarette. The time in seclusion varies, but when it is felt that you have settled down you are let out.

But when I first went into this room, it wasn't like that. My story is about the room I first went into in the mental hospital at the tender age of sixteen.

The Room

by Toby Adams [2]

'Wake up, Son. Hey, wake up. '

'What!'

'Wake up. We are going to take you to the doctor. We're going with Uncle. Get out of bed.'

'How long have I been asleep?'

'Three days.'

'It was that stuff that the doctor gave me that knocked me out.'

'It was running around on the bloody streets that knocked you out. Now hurry up, we are going to another doctor. You're sick and we need to do something about it. Get some warm clothes on and something to eat and we're off.'

I had been running ragged for the last couple of weeks. In an exhausted state. I was taken to a GP who recommended that I be placed in an institution. I then was given an injection that made me unconscious for three days. I was then taken to a psychiatrist who diagnosed me as having a mental disorder. Then I was taken to Kingseat Hospital.

I had no idea what was going on. I thought it was a great adventure. Coupled with the fantasy world that I was in, I did not know that this would be a turning point in my life, and I was entering a life that would change me for ever.

Boy what a neat ride, I wonder where we are going now? I'd never been to this place before. Look at all the buildings all over the place and the people wandering around. They all look spaced out. Mind you, I feel pretty spaced out myself.

As we pulled up to the hospital I had no idea what this place was. The hospital was situated in huge grounds. The wards were two-storey buildings called villas that were separated from each other. It had a football, soccer and hockey field. From what I remember, it had at least ten villas and a huge gym hall with an outdoor swimming pool. On the other side of the grounds there was an indoor heated pool, a bowling green and tennis court. The main building was administration, this also had a ward. It had long-term and short-term patients.

'Yes. Bring your son in here, Mr Adams. You can go into the lounge, Toby. We'll be with you in a minute.'

I walk into the lounge, and look around. The people look strange.

The room was strange. The whole place was strange. I got to the window and took off! In those days I could move. I cleared the footpath in one leap and was off at full tilt with no idea where I was going. Next minute, one person was behind me giving chase, then two, then another. Boy, could they move! But I was way ahead. Then bang! I ran into someone in front of me. I fought like hell but there were too many of them. Then I was picked up and taken to the room.

They gave me an injection. Stripped me down and put pj's on me. In this room was a mattress, a blanket, a pillow and a pot to do your business on. It had a giant door and a shutter over the window. I don't know how long I was out for but it was dark outside and the light was on when I woke up.

Where the hell am I! Wow, that's right!

'Hey! Is there anyone out there? Hey, you bastards, let me out!' Man, I've got to stand up. Boy, I'm cold.

'Hey! Is there anyone out there?' Boy, I feel woozy. I wonder what that pot's for? You're kidding!

'Hey let me out of this place!' Man I'm cold! Bugger this. I'm getting out.

To explain what sort of high I was on is hard to do. But when I made the decision to get out I went 'hard'. I went up to the door and smashed at it with my fists. I looked up and saw someone looking through the small slit in the door. I got up, went for the back wall then went hard out for the door. *Bang!* The person moved away from the door. I got up and did it again and again, all the time yelling, 'Let me out! Let me out!'

Totally exhausted and sore, I crawled back to the bed. It was about this time the door opened. Four or five staff came in checked me over, cleaned up the place, checked the pot and gave me more medication. With that done they left, with me powerless to follow, saying under my breath, 'Let me out. Let me out. Let me out.'

When I woke up I found myself still in this nightmare. I was hoping it was all a bad dream. But it wasn't.

Sore, tired and cold, the door opened. The staff came in and asked me if I was all right. I couldn't say much, or do anything, so they brought in breakfast. I ate a little, then they gave me more medication and left, with me wishing I could, too.

I remember sitting there looking at the walls, crying with this great hopelessness in my heart. I then started singing. I think I felt that if I could not escape the room, I was going to escape with my mind. I started to sing songs that I grew up with. Maori ones, the latest songs of the times. Even Christmas songs. It felt good.

Then I heard yelling and laughing at the door. I walked up to it and there were women there who I thought were patients. They would yell then laugh and weren't making any sense, but then nothing in this place did. I looked at the door and something was coming underneath it. I then realised they were peeing from the other side. I went nuts.

Bang! bang! I hit the door as hard and fast as I could, using my hands, feet, head, and body, with all my strength and willpower, yelling all the time, 'Let me out! Let me out! Let me out!'

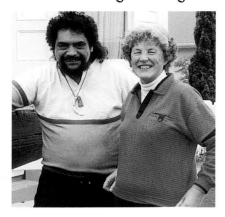

I would like to thank Kath Algie for the support and the Christian Fellowship her and her family have given me.

I don't remember much of what happened over the next couple of days. They did feed me, and I did get an extra blanket. I was highly medicated and finally did calm down. But I did go for the door a few more times.

I must say, I was out of control, and in no way do I blame the staff or anyone at the time, for putting me in there. I was a young man who had an illness, and who did not know what was happening to him. Please remember, I was at the young age of sixteen. I now have a lot of insight and experience that help me deal with this illness, and also have the ability to help others cope with their illnesses.

I did eventually get out of the room, and it was a start of a life that has been challenging and exciting. It is a life that I did not plan to have, but adversity has made me stronger.

Everyone has pain at some time in their lives that they must deal with. I help others, and that helps me deal with mine. To my family who never once abandoned me I give great thanks and also to my friends who have stood by me over the years.

Also to the various medical people who have helped me, Thank you. These are the tools that have helped me cope with this illness.

Postscript

I am now working closer with the consumer movement and have taken on board Christianity. I am to be baptised before this book is published.

I have to be honest with me, says

Lynda Delamore

Lynda is forty-eight and is married to Vincent Reidy and is, with him, a co-director of Point Erin House, Terwindle Lodge and Safet House in Herne Bay, Auckland. She is the mother of two daughters.

I have just really got on with my life and picked the pieces up and moved forward. Often I've felt I'd love to write a book myself. I'd love to tell my story. This is a really good positive thing and I'm excited about it.

But I'm also anxious as I don't often talk about this period of my life or how I feel about my experiences. When somebody is actually interested, it is a bit of a shock. I've paid lots of money for people to be very bored by it, and that's been no help whatsoever. So that's really why I'm working in mental health. There are a lot of good people in this field, and we've just got to get our stories out and heard.

My husband, Vin, and I operate two Level III and one Level IV psychiatric rehab homes.[1] I hate that terminology, but there's really no other way to put it. I worked in the drug and alcohol field for a number of years, and a social worker friend of mine took me along to a barbeque here and it fascinated me. I fell in love with the people. They were so clear. Yes, they were unwell and they were very heavily medicated, but they were just themselves and I was fascinated by it. It was very 'rest-homey', and I knew that different things could be done for these people. So I came to work here and was really excited about it.

Then out of the blue I met Vincent. He was at a stage in his life where he had been made redundant and hadn't worked for three years. We were obviously looking for something, apart from each other. And it seemed to be the right thing. So that's how we ended up working in this field. Now I think, *Well, it was meant to be, and we were meant to be here.*

In fact, I'd realised that, while I had dealt with my drug and alcohol issues and could easily talk about those, I'd never spoken to people about my experiences in psychiatric hospitals. Maybe that was my fear about going to work in this area, and I really had to analyse my own feelings. And I'm quite happy to cry about this – I think it's very healthy.

My own life was a bloody shambles. I had been married three times, and been through all sorts of experiences. But I had reached the stage where I thought, *You've worked so bloody hard.* I guess at that point I was starting to think, *Maybe it is time to grow up, Lynda, and get responsible.* I mean, I've always felt like I'm visiting this planet and that I've been on the fucking outskirts of it all my life. Excuse me swearing, but I rather like that word – it sort of helps.

I'm the only girl in a family of three – I've got an older brother and a younger brother. My mother married the wrong man and stayed with him for us children. My dad was alcoholic and my mum was a pill freak. Dad died at thirty-six of a heart attack and Mum was killed in an accident when I was nineteen. My younger brother, who was only fourteen at the time, was seriously injured in it and I came back from Australia to look after him.

That was when my life went down. I was using alcohol. I'd been singing in a band in Australia and getting on with my life. Alcohol hadn't affected me too much at that stage. I used to get pissed and get a hangover and make a big Joe of myself but, you know, all of a sudden I had all this responsibility.

I chose to deal with it by drinking. By the time I was twenty-two, I was pregnant, I was looking after my brother, I was in a state house and then I met my first husband, who was a ratbag. He was in prison more often than not, and I spent most of our married life going to Paremoremo every Saturday with two little children. So all of this was going on in my life. No wonder I was a drunk!

It was during that time I realised I really did feel like an alien. One night, when I was really really down (my daughter was about ten months), I took some pills and I also loaded her bottle with pills. But I didn't give it to her. I sort of lay in bed with her for ages. Then a friend rang up, and he sensed something was wrong. He turned up in a taxi and raced me into Auckland Hospital.

I ended up in Ward 10, the psychiatric ward, being told by everybody that I was mad. I went in there looking for help, but I couldn't really understand that system.

The second day I was there, a woman of fifty-eight was admitted. The psychiatrist got me to sit in on her initial interview. I could never really work out why they did that. Still, even to this day, I don't understand it. I mean, were they trying to work out if *I* had an alcohol problem? I wish they had asked me. I would have told them, *Yes I do*. But nobody ever asked me, which really intrigued me. They used to have a community meeting every morning, and the woman was a bit anti-social and didn't want to go. Neither did I, really. But the next morning I was sitting on her bed and said to her, *Come on, let's just go. Let's give them what they want, you know, we'll be well trained.* And she said, *I'm not fucking going there*. The next thing these (I think there were about four) burly bloody nurses came flying down, grabbed her off the bed, took her away and put this jacket thing on her. She was screaming. I've never been so upset in all my life. Then this sister came back and said to me, *I know you might think that's a bit rough, but it's for her own good*. They carted her off to Kingseat. And I never saw her again. I just couldn't come to terms with that, you know. I made the decision I was going to leave. And I did.

Then I had about four more years of drinking. I *did* try to address the issue. I went to my own doctor who worked at the drug and alcohol unit at Kingseat. I used to go to him and say, *Oh Christ, my life's in a mess*. I was on Valium by this stage. And he said, *Look Lynda, people respond to stress in different ways and that's what you're doing*. Well, you know, that's all very well. But at that point I did need more awareness about the problem.

So I just went on taking more pills and drinking more alcohol and wandering around the planet wondering what it was all about. Hearing people

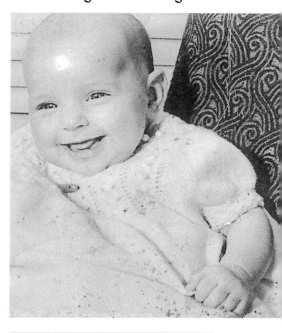

This is me at about nine months old.

say they'd had a hard life and thinking, *Well shit, I would love to tell you* my *story*.

Anyway, I decided that I was going to buy my own home as a solo parent. I was on the domestic purposes benefit and I thought, *I'm not going to bloody well live like a pauper all my life. I deserve better than this.* So I struggled and pushed and pulled and finally did it.

But I was still drinking and my doctor referred me to Papakura day hospital. I went there for one day and they asked me to draw a picture of a tree. I spent eight hours there and I thought, *What's this all about?* You know, I was still grieving for my mother. Nobody ever asked me how I felt about this.

So anyway, I went back to my doctor and I said, *Look, this isn't working, I can't go there and draw trees and try and relate that to my life, you know. I'm in a mess, I need help.* Anyway, he suggested that I go to Kingseat, as a voluntary patient.

I'm sitting there. The psychiatrist interviews me. I talk to him about my mother dying and the hassle I've got in my life and it's all gone to pieces. And he says to me, *Do you know your mother is dead?* I say, *I know she's dead, I've just been telling you – what the fuck's wrong with you?*

I mean, you know, there may have been relevant reasons for what he was doing. Then he wanted to get my family involved and I said, *I've been telling you that my two brothers are so separate from me at the moment, the last thing I want them to know is that I am in a nut-house. Don't do this to me.* And I started getting very distrustful then, because I was quite separate from my family at that point.

So, anyway, we went and sat in a bloody circle and we had to pretend that somebody dropped 50 cents in front of us. There were about twenty of us really well-trained little animals walking around the room, people tapping each other on the shoulder and giving back the 50 cents. Not me! I put it in my pocket and ran away!

I just did everything I could to be disruptive. And I was getting grief for this. They put me in a side ward. I suppose it was the assessment area.

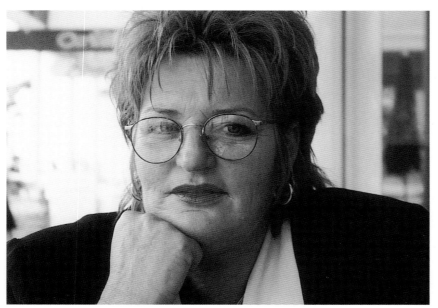

Photograph by Julie Leibrich

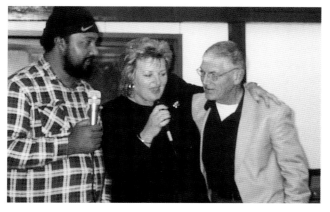

A Karaoke Night at Point Erin House.

They shoved me in a room with a young kid, bless her, who was eighteen. Her father had left home and she had cracked up, hadn't slept for days, and they were knocking her out with pills. She wouldn't go to sleep and all night long she was calling out, *I want my Daddy.*

By three o'clock in the morning I said, *For fuck's sake, get in here with me.* And I got her into bed with me. And I'm patting her head, while she falls asleep in my arms.

Meanwhile, the woman next door was talking about her dead brother. I mean, I knew nothing about voices. And come the second night they were going to put me back in this room, and I said, *I am not going. All I want to do is see my children. I don't care what you say about me, I want to see my children.* I left, but I had to promise I would come back. So I left my passion-killer there, which is my favourite nightie. I wonder who ended up with it?

Then my journey *really* took off into alcoholism. Yes, I really went down. I remember the exact moment when I crossed over from abusing alcohol to being alcoholic. It was almost a decision. I'd fought for everything in my life, like I'd fought for that house. And I looked around that house and I thought, *You've got it all kid, but you still feel bad.* And I remember that moment to this day.

I was a binge drinker – the hardest person to get through to because you can really kid yourself that you don't need it. So I'd get on a binge for two or three days, then I'd pull myself together and get on with it. And then another binge.

So I sat back after looking at this totally disastrous life and thought, *Well I suppose I could say it's Mum and Dad's fault.* But I have a spiritual concept of karma. I believe that I chose my mum and dad to teach me the lessons I needed to know in life from their mistakes. Hopefully I'd learnt from their

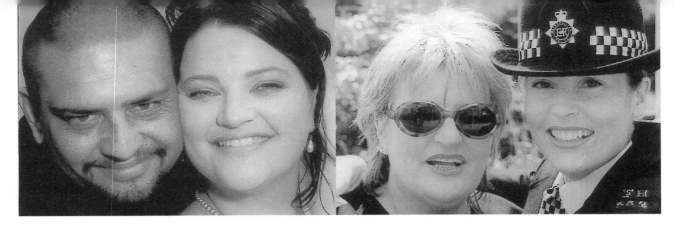

I'm very proud of my daughters. Toni is a policewoman in London, and Cerise, along with her husband David, just about runs our organisation!

mistakes. But then I said to myself, *I've not only made their mistakes; now I'm creating my own.*

So I rented my house out and moved up to Henderson because I wanted to change my life. I was only there six months and one day I put my kids in the car after drinking large, large amounts of wine and I had a car accident. I nearly killed my children, and for me that was *it*.

I decided I just couldn't go on like this or I'd shoot myself. I went to AA. I got into recovery, which I'm still in today. I had to *deal* with my life. I tell you what kept me sober for the first six months. I used to get all these negative thoughts in my head. The only thing that really ever made sense to me in AA was the 'Serenity Prayer':

God, grant me the serenity to accept the things I cannot change, the courage to change the things I can and the wisdom to know the difference.

I used to just say that prayer, and say that prayer, and say it, say it, say it, and I wouldn't say anything else. I see now it's a thought-stopping process, but that's what I used and it worked. I've got it all over my house. People walk into my house and think I'm bloody religious. It's even on my mirror. But I needed to do more with my life than just go to AA. I hadn't been through all this to end up not feeling good about me. So I decided I was going to do some voluntary work and I went off to the Salvation Army and to Social Detox and worked there.[2] I got on with people and decided I'd like to do the CIT addiction study certificate.[3] I completed that and got a job in the field with community addiction services.

I've been recovering since then. Actually I don't like the word *recovery*. I have thought long and hard about this, and I've thought long and hard about my experiences. What is recovery for me? (And we'll use that word for want of a better word at the moment.) It's about this: *I have to be honest with* me.

I *do* have a mouth, and because I *do* challenge people, it's got me into a lot of crap in my life. I've learnt who it matters to be honest with. Once upon a time I would have seen that as manipulative, but I don't now. I see it as being smart. I think recovery for me is about getting smart.

This planet is about them and us, whether we like it or not. I am intuitive, and I trust that and I know myself. I know when I'm getting stretched by things. I know I have to look after myself – like remembering to say HALT, when you're Hungry, Angry, Lonely or Tired. They're just the basic principles.

I protect myself mentally. I just put a steel shield around myself mentally. I mean it's a metaphysical thing, and it works for me. It stops me from responding to the unreasonableness my feelings allow me to get into sometimes. But it's about me protecting me, really.

I feel I've done amazingly well. But I've had to be a strong woman. Even bolshie. I'm a 'get on with it, stop giving me bullshit, let's deal with it' kind of person. I'm clear. I realised this when I worked in the drug and alcohol field, because I was *challenging*. If I was a guy that would be totally acceptable. My behaviour would seem tame in a man. So I believe women have a real battle.

The relationships that I've really had to work on are with women. This has been difficult for me. It's easy with men, because I work through my sexuality. I'm at ease with my sexuality and so I wear it lovingly – it's quite nice. But when women sense that, they don't like it. And that's been difficult. My women friends often make comments about my weight. It's all about self image. It's really interesting how people react to me depending on where my weight is at. Just the way they look at you. I mean it's subtle, really. It's not overt. That's discrimination.

I don't think that my experiences with alcohol or even psychiatric units make me special, but I think the way in which I survive does. And I'm proud of this. I mean I look at what Vin and I are doing now. Vin's an academic and I'm a people person. I think we're a good combination in that he's got the head stuff and I've got the heart stuff.

It isn't about being special or having a special understanding. This is about being human and treating people as human beings, not as cases. When we work in an area like this, I believe we have a total duty, a responsibility, to treat people as human beings.

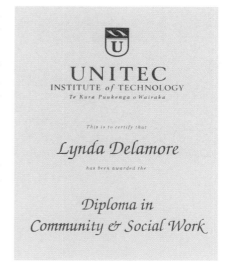

Lynda's diploma of Social Work

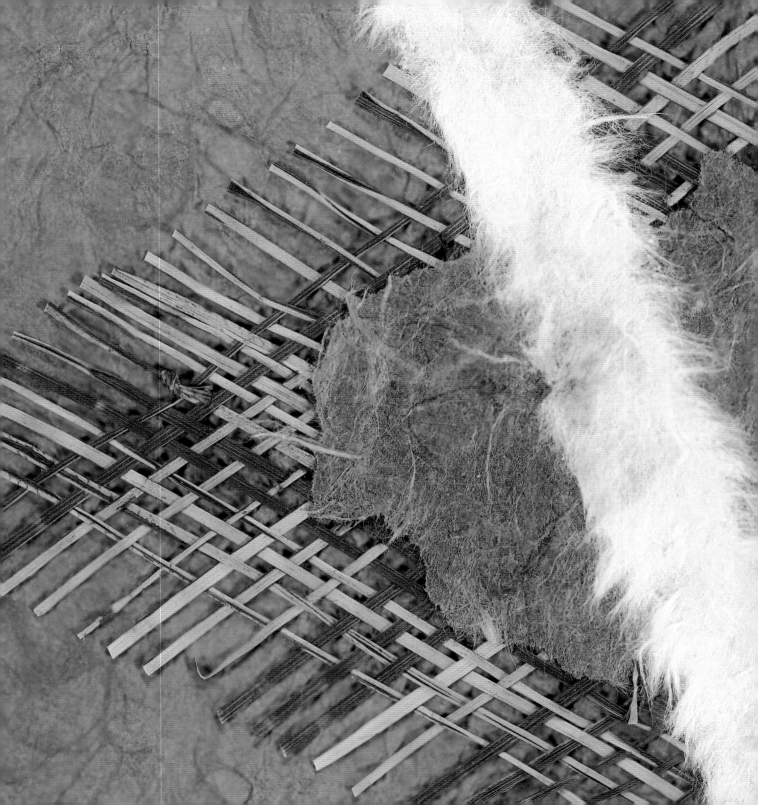

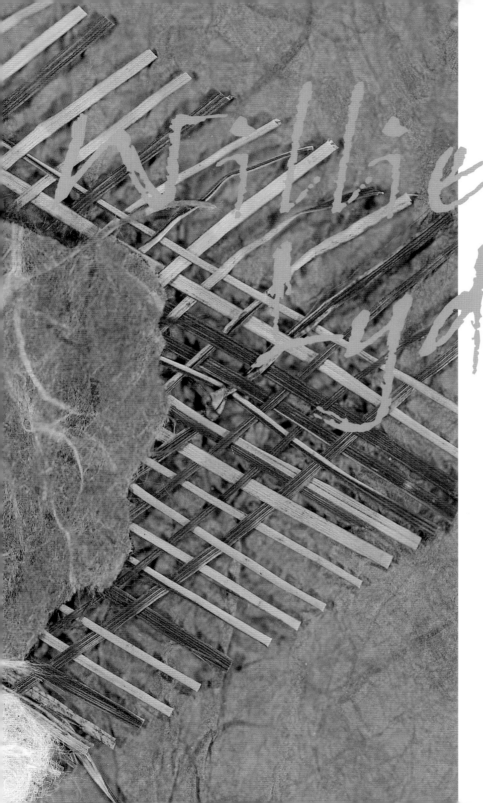

I've come a long way,
says

Willie Hyden

Willie is twenty-eight and lives in Auckland in one of the houses that Lynda and Vince run. He works in a factory called Industrial Enterprises and he likes Karaoke, drawing, making model cars and buying clothes.

I come from a big family. I'm half Irish and half Tongan. When I was a little boy my father died and I lived with my mum and my sister. I used to come back from school and get changed and go to my uncle's place.

I liked school because I could draw pictures there. But I didn't learn to read or write. I had some

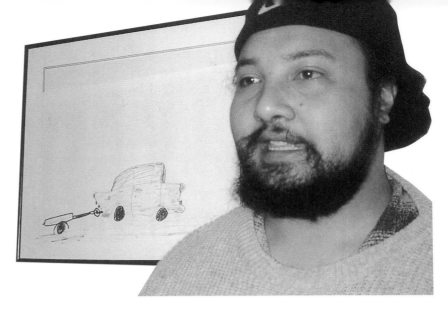

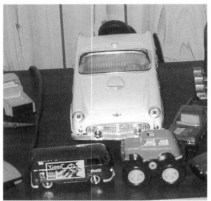

I love model cars.

difficulty at school. I sometimes got into boys' fights. And I got into trouble three times for nicking my dad's cigarettes after school. But I was a good boy.

But I wasn't happy when I was teenager and started to live on the streets. It was a hard life. I didn't have enough to eat and I slept on the street. I used to sniff glue and paint. I liked to sniff red paint best because it reminded me of a round tin of chocolates that my Dad had. Plus I used to drink a lot of beer. Sometimes I felt like I was aggressive with people.

When I was sixteen I was admitted to Carrington because I was really unwell and tried to hurt somebody.[1] Even though the hospital is closed now, I still don't like going near it because a lot of bad things happened there.

I lived in a few hostels for a while, but I still wasn't well. And when I was twenty-two, I got into trouble with the police and went to jail. I was living in a flat with another guy and he assaulted me and took my money off me. Every time I got paid from the Social Welfare he tried to rob the money from my pockets and spend it on booze. He didn't want me in the flat with him, and every day he was giving me stuff he stole. He actually kept on coming to my room at night and taking my money – about twenty bucks – and spending it on cans of beer. This guy tried to get me really drunk. He gave me about four cans. I got pissed and he tried to slam me, but he slammed another bloke instead. I had a fight with the guy and I was out on the street.

I went to a mate's place and he was half pissed and I stuffed his crowbar underneath my jumper and walked up the hill. I remember I went into a church centre and I got a bit angry because they wouldn't serve me. Then the cops came and arrested me and put the handcuffs on my hands and took me into downtown Central. They took me in the police car. I remember. When they had those Falcons. I remember this cop pulled up and said to me, *Right fella we're taking you down the station.*

When I first walked in, they put me in a cell, with no clothes on. I was bloody naked. The time came to take off my shoes and they said to me, *We don't care. We've got your clothes. You can go to sleep in the blanket.*

They took down my fingerprints and just chucked me in the cell for the night. They gave me chips and sausages about midnight. They were nasty to me because when I asked them for cigarettes they didn't want to give me any. Half of the time I was banging on the door. I said to the cop, *I need some toilet paper to wipe my arse.*

They sent me to Court and then to jail. Then they just sent me to Kingseat, and then they sent me to Kauri Unit in the Mason Clinic.[2] When I'd been at the Mason Clinic about twelve weeks, they sent me out to Kahikatea.[3] They had an action note from my lawyer to the police and they had to let me go. And I came to live here.

I've lived here for seven years. I have my own room. I like living here. Because I can move around lot, you know. You can do your washing and I can help wipe the tables and sweep the floors. Plus I got my own money in my bank, and I can actually walk up the road and get it.

I can talk to Lynda about things, and I'm doing a reading course. It's better than the streets and better than in hospital. It's a free life and I can go and buy things, like clothes and CDs. And I've got a few friends

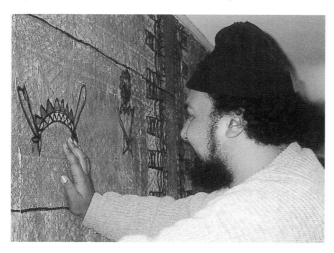

A reminder of my culture.

here. Sometimes I get a bit upset if the guys annoy me for cigarettes. But I talk to Lynda and she listens to me. She looks out for me.

I met Lynda when she first came here. And she said to me, *You've been a naughty boy!* Because when I first met her I had five hats, about five shirts, and three jackets on, because I didn't trust people. So I didn't want to leave my clothes in my room.

Now, I only get really angry sometimes. I get on with people easier now. Lynda told me that when she last spoke to my sister she was really proud of me because I had grown up. My sister said that now I would tell her off about doing things she did wrong but she isn't scared any more. I trust some people more. Just friends. Even that guy who took the money from me. We actually shook hands and I made up friends with him.

I go to work now, at Industrial Enterprises. I go with my mates. I work not far from the Mason Clinic, not far from Carrington. I help the boss to sellotape the boxes and put them onto the pallets. And he tells me I'm a good man, I'm doing a good job.

I have lunch up in the canteen. I'm one of the workers. I usually get a Coke and a pie, and I go up to the top and help myself to a cup of tea and sit on the chair. I go over with one of the guys and have a few games on the pool table.

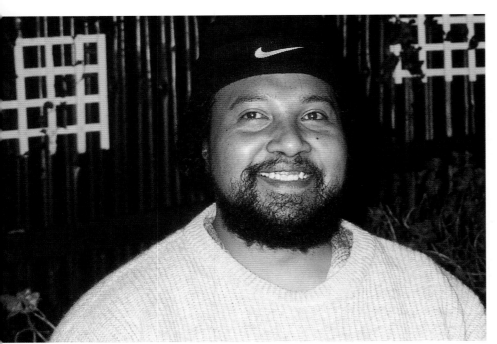

I get on with guys. I have some friends in the factory. And if the guys have arguments, I try to help out and make them stop.

I've got a girlfriend. I met her at work. She's nice and pretty. We're only friends. I don't want to get into a relationship with her because I don't want to end up getting kids with her. I'm worried in case I might not be a really good man to her. It's just something that I have to work out.

I try to take care of myself, so I take my medication, myself, every day. If I didn't have my medication I wouldn't be 100 per cent well. These pills are there to make me feel well.

My life's pretty settled. I go home every second weekend to stay with my family. I go to church when I go home. I stay with my uncle and my mum and my sister and I like it. But my mum can't have me there all the time because there's people out on the streets that don't trust me and wouldn't treat me fair. And it's hard to get a job near there. And I love my job in Industrial Enterprises.

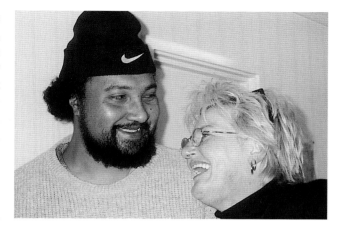

Me and Lynda.

I enjoy most things in life, even the shower in the mornings and going for a walk up the road. Sometimes I do my washing, and on the weekend I get up really late for breakfast. And I like to sing on the Karaoke.

I am good at painting. I like to paint another coat on that chair over there so every time someone sits on it they're going to get paint on their bums! I mean, I'm not a real artist but I can draw. I draw boats, mountains, trucks, cars, bridges, you know – those bridges that have those tall lights. I like to use colour felt-tips to draw pictures because I like colour.

I am learning to write properly now, on a course. When I first started to write, one of the things I remember was my hand wasn't too good. My hand was shaking. But now I'm trying to write my name really straight. I'm trying to write properly and draw properly.

Mary McKearny, who used to work here, used to call me Magic-Man. Every time she visits she still calls me Magic-Man. Because when I first came here I wasn't really 100 per cent. You know, I wasn't really good.

My life's really changed. I've come a long way from when I lived in that flat to here.

What I think is, I try my best. I do my work here that has to be done. You know, I do the best I can in life. I try not to put people down but I stand up for myself.

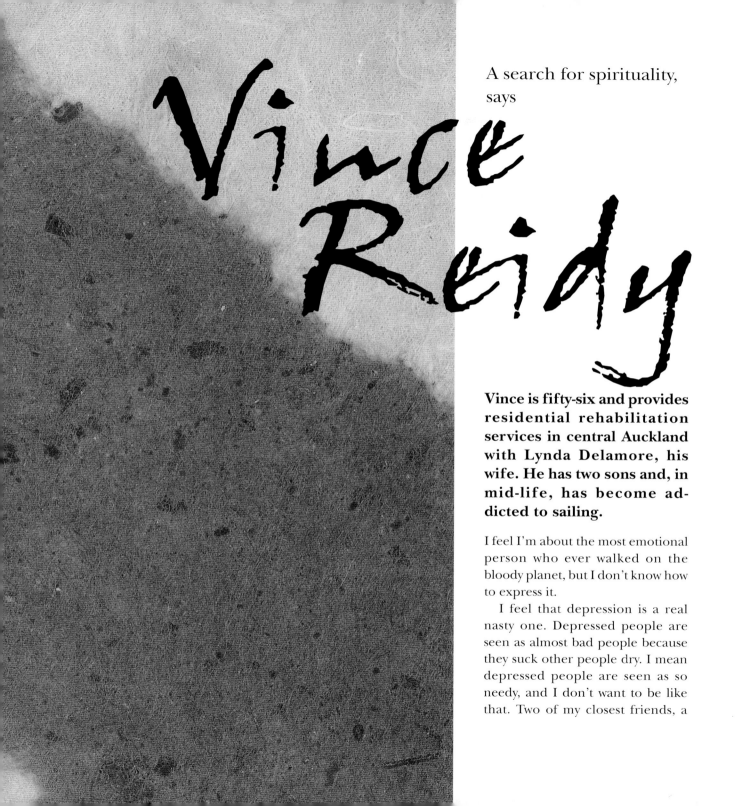

A search for spirituality, says

Vince Reidy

Vince is fifty-six and provides residential rehabilitation services in central Auckland with Lynda Delamore, his wife. He has two sons and, in mid-life, has become addicted to sailing.

I feel I'm about the most emotional person who ever walked on the bloody planet, but I don't know how to express it.

I feel that depression is a real nasty one. Depressed people are seen as almost bad people because they suck other people dry. I mean depressed people are seen as so needy, and I don't want to be like that. Two of my closest friends, a married couple whom I love very dearly, are content to have drinks, eat and chat and laugh with me but don't let me 'indulge' in what I feel deep down, feelings which can produce tears on occasions. It's the advice, the common sense advice, the knee-jerk advice, the boys out fishing, the 'just pull your bloody finger out and stop feeling sorry for yourself'. That's the discrimination about depression.

I even discriminate against myself about being depressed. I've got a kind of stereotype about depression in my head. It's been in the family. I'm sure my mother had depression. I can remember her crying over the back fence talking to the neighbours. One of her brothers suicided way back in about the 1930s, and that's come down as a family story. But Irish families didn't really talk about these things. I didn't want to be like that so I've got a whole lot of messages in my head saying, *You don't want to be one of those depressed sort of serious, bloody dour kind of people!*

It's like an emotional straitjacket this stuff, and I've only just started to live free from it over the last three or four years. What you're looking at here is a very, very emotionally 'young' journey in an older physical frame – you know, going on for twenty, thirty, forty years – that's what I'm trying to describe.

My parents were third-generation New Zealanders from an Irish background. My father was one of a generation that was actually more Irish than the Irish. They identified themselves as Irish even though they spoke with a New Zealand accent. Being Catholic, being a Mick, was their cultural identity. And there was significant discrimination against them in Dunedin in those days when I was at school.

My mother was over-protective about me, and I was trying to be, you know, a strong bloke in this male rugby school set-up. And I actually enjoyed school because it was an escape, a freedom, a vehicle to get away from home. Really, with puberty, the beautiful possibilities. Wonderful!

And I bloody well blew it by going to the seminary, instead of just going up to the other end of town and taking a flat and going to Otago University and being normal. I very stupidly did 'the right thing' – I've spent most of my life doing the 'right' thing. The seminary was just awful. All I can say is that that was where I got into life as a pretty bloody dull business.

So I grew up totally in that Irish Catholic sub-culture and spent eight years studying for the Catholic priesthood. My mother died in my seventh year, and in the twelve months or so after that I became utterly depressed and unable to function.

I left the seminary determined not to go home and live with Dad in a

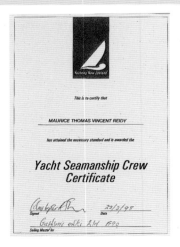

One of my greatest achievements so far – it means self reliance and courage to go out onto the sea alone.

This is to certify that

MAURICE THOMAS VINCENT REIDY

has attained the necessary standard and is awarded the

Yacht Seamanship Crew Certificate

sort of Steptoe and Son set-up, so I moved to Wellington and went straight into a homosexual relationship. I had no idea it was that or going to be that, when it was happening. I was a 'mummy's boy' and essentially seduced by an early-middle-aged man. Looking back now, I realise that I was in a homosexual relationship, however implicit, even earlier, with the local curate when I was in my teens.

Anyway, I realised that I had got into a very bad relationship in Wellington when I read a book which was a bit cute on psychology and deception (I think it was *The Magus*).[1] For two or three years I lived this sort of life, and every time I went out with a girl he found a reason for her not to be suitable. I kind of bought that and went along with it, until my first wife came along and he started the same sort of thing about her. For the first time I could see that this was all a manipulation. So I ended the relationship and really bounced out of it into my first marriage.

Then my wife and I went to London. That was a terribly depressing bloody time. I just hated it; we had no money. I hated living in the big smoke, just being one of millions on Victoria Street. I know it's glamorous when you're on a visit, but to me, living there, I just felt totally trapped by it. I felt like a fly pinned to the wall.

That lasted only two or three years and I came home without the PhD I had read for at the London School of Economics. I taught sociology to medical students in the Department of Psychological Medicine at the Wellington Clinical School for six or seven years and I hated that place, too. I felt like a nude in church! I just felt totally out of place, no clear role – I couldn't work out what I was supposed to be doing. In the end I just couldn't do it any more.

My whole approach to what I think is my quite definite emotional instability, if I can call it that, is that I made every effort to compensate for it and hide it.

It wasn't until I did some personal development workshops when my first marriage split in 1992 that I suddenly discovered that there was a whole bunch of ordinary people who were just like me. The great middle class was well represented on that first weekend and they actually accepted me as having had experiences very similar to their own. Really it was the first time, perhaps in decades, perhaps since school, that I ever received permission to talk about the things that had made me think I was very, very crazy, and very out of whack emotionally.

There have been several bad times. I suppose on a scale of one to ten, my first marriage split was about nine-and-a-half out of ten bad. I ended up

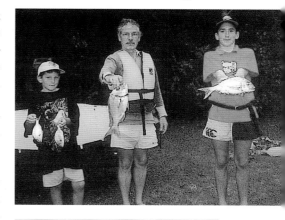

My sons, Frederick and Christopher. Hari Nui, Campbells Beach, 1996–97.

flatting on my own. At the same time I went through a redundancy, and was conscious of my age, and I'd lost my two sons; well, that's how it felt, anyway.

I'm sure it was clinical depression, but I suppose I've always tried to deny that there was anything really wrong. I didn't want to ever have a name put on it. But I did spend two or three years crying, and actually still do and can very easily, and I think that is depression. It is an emotional problem of flatness.

I remember experiencing despair. Suicide was never really an option, but I did think about it because life did seem pretty pointless. I had no concrete hope during those months and years. It was just a matter of keeping on keeping on, grasping positive ideas from all sorts of sources and discovering for the first time an inner strength.

I read a reasonable amount of the personal development stuff, I went on just about every workshop that was available around Auckland, and mixed in what used to be called, and probably still are called, New Age circles. I just derived a positivity from that. In fact, I got into what I now consider to be some quite wacky ideas. I actually finished up in a millennialist religious cult. For twelve months or more, I trotted along there once a week, or a fortnight, and did meditations and that kept me going. That was preceded by doing some primal therapy, again looking for some key to unlock it all.

I came back a bit to a more conservative therapy and did long-term counselling over a year or two with an ACC registered counsellor to deal with some emotional abuse issues around my mother. So that's respectable

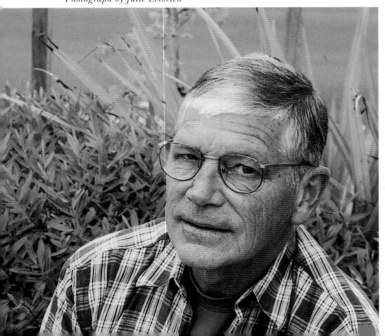

Photograph by Julie Leibrich

stuff. (Much of the stuff I did earlier was actually not 'respectable' at all. You know, what some people might call 'wacky'.) I did the counselling because I had discovered, as a result of introspection, that there was (and I don't want to over-dramatise it) definitely emotional abuse in my upbringing by my parents, and I did some counselling long term over that. I've got a terrible feeling this sounds so trivial, but family dynamics can have a hell of a big effect on the way you operate in adult relationships.

As I say it to you, it sounds so nice and respectable – middle-class workshops and so on. But in fact it was a very painful, grubby, dirty, mucky business getting in there and going down into it and then coming to terms with it and coming out again.

I had spent the best part of two decades in an unhappy marriage which I did not recognise as unhappy. I thought that was as good as it got. And here's where I take responsibility. I had somehow invited and allowed being put down and controlled by my ex-wife, in a way which did her no good either, of course. That was the basic dynamic and I spent twenty years learning how to lose my self-esteem. For whatever reason, that's what I spent the twenty years doing – becoming a non-person.

The last five or six years of that marriage (we had a ten-acre lifestyle block) I lived out the back in a pretty run-down shed. It was not quite as bad as, but a bit like, that guy in Dunedin, the father in the Bain case. I was living outside in squalor, and my ex-wife and my two boys lived in the house. I spent a lot of time using alcohol – I don't think to a worrying extent, but my big consolation at night was to sit on the back verandah and have two or three cans of lager and that made it all bearable. Then I had a meal after my ex-wife and the boys had gone to bed and then I crashed out in the shed out the back. Each morning I would don the corporate uniform – the dark suit – and spend the rest of the day making every effort to be bright-eyed and bushy-tailed as a corporate trainer.

The point I want to make is that I spent those twenty years not looking at any issues in my life at all. I thought that what you had to do (typically male thing) was get out there and be successful, and for me that meant in a corporate situation. Climb to the top and get the company car and all that stuff. Funnily enough, the whole career thing came to an end at the same time as the marriage.

As I said there was a redundancy – in fact that was the third redundancy. The whole corporate thing didn't work for me. I worked very hard at it, but somehow it just didn't work. So a whole lot of things had come to a great full stop at the age of just on fifty. And it was like, *Where the hell do I go from here?*

At that point I met Lynda. I had done three years' hard bloody work going right down into the 'what's it all about'. Depression, despair, the whole bit – looking in every direction for therapy, philosophy, religion, spirituality, you name it … I mean, I've sat at the feet of American Indians. I've done the lot.

I guess my learning is that I wouldn't want to go to a psychiatrist (as I had done during my time teaching at the Clinical School). I would rather do it another way. I'd rather listen to somebody who treats it as an educational challenge rather than an illness. That's a distinction that I found very useful, because I never had to consider myself ill. There's no label. I

Lead, Kindly Light

Lead, kindly Light, amid the
encircling gloom,
Lead Thou me on!
The night is dark, and I am far from
home –
Lead Thou me on!
Keep thou my feet; I do not ask to see
The distant scene – one step enough
for me.
I was not ever thus, nor prayed that
thou
Shouldst lead me on.
I loved to choose and see my path;
but now,
Lead Thou me on!
I loved the garish day, and, spite of
fears,
Pride ruled my will: remember not
past years.
So long Thy power hath blessed me,
sure it still
Will lead me on,
O'er moor and fen, o'er crag and
torrent, till
The night is gone;
And with the morn those angle faces
smile
Which I have loved long since, and
lost awhile.

Cardinal John Henry Newman
(1808–1890)

I love the universal mysticism of this man, who suffered within his own tradition and went well beyond it.

only had to consider myself as having a lot to learn. Also my experiences were, in a way, validated. They were valuable.

It's not the shit that you get into, it's the way you react to it. I found this so positive and so refreshing. It doesn't make it any easier but it does enable you to keep a kind of optimism, or a kind of a sense that it's all got a meaning, in a way.

There were a lot of really quite well-thought-of courses going on around Auckland in those days. There was an outfit over in Newmarket called Key Seminars. They ran a seminar, a weekender called Turning Point. I did that weekend and thoroughly enjoyed it. You got the opportunity to do a little bit of pillow thumping, and a little bit of screaming, and a little bit of talking about it, and a little bit of sort of spirituality. In fact, for me, personal development is really about searching for, and developing, a valid personal spirituality.

What I took from those New Age courses was that I didn't have to be some kind of permanent renegade Catholic. I just divorced myself from it and cut my emotional ties with it, and got in touch with more personal spirituality than I ever could in a structured system. This made me realise that spirituality is far more than Catholicism. I think underlying all of my life is a search for spirituality. I now regard myself as a true catholic (without the capital C) in my spirituality.

Underlying most of these things, it seems to me, is a kind of Eastern spirituality. I think it seems to come from Hinduism and Buddhism, rather than anywhere else. One of the ideas I've kept is that we're here just to learn lessons. I'm also open to the possibility that there is some kind of a cycle of birth and rebirth. Primal therapy can take you down this path.

But, I don't think that kind of connection and emotional openness and comfort has been easy for me. I don't think I have, by any means, achieved quick resolution, or closure, because I'm inclined to go 'left-brain' all the time. I'm a bit withdrawn from emotional stuff. I tend to operate pretty analytically most of the time. I've just got to let go of control, and I find it really scary. Because when I let go of control I just feel as if I become an emotional jellyfish and a big blob, and that doesn't feel very comfortable for me. It doesn't feel very *male*. It's quite scary, and I feel it. I've probably still got to deal with it, I guess.

I learnt self-control at a very young age and Catholicism certainly reinforced it.

I can remember riding along in a little Ford Prefect with sunny little bubble headlights, you know, those tall Ford Prefects. Sitting in the back.

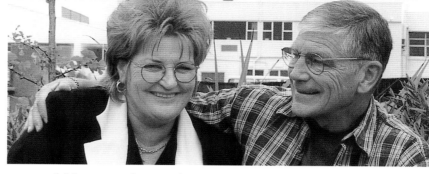

With my wife, Lynda.

Parents in the front. Sunday drive – which always turned to shit because they always had a row. Just thinking, *Well, I can control this*, just sitting there. It was like I made a decision somewhere at the age of seven or eight, that I could keep out of it by controlling it. I would fantasise about my model boat, or whatever it was that I liked to do. Fantasise about when I was going to listen to the radio, or what I was going to eat for tea. It was like a switching off. So my experience of emotions has always been that emotions fuck you up. I'm not justifying it; I'm saying that that's probably the theme.

Isn't it strange, though, that one would go through life avoiding anything to do with social work or therapising people. Trying to play it straight, trying to be an academic. Trying to be a corporate high flier. Trying to do all the straight things, having a house in the suburbs and even a lifestyle block. Doing all that, just chatting over the barbecue, and doing all the right sort of things.

Then really, not being forced to, but going right back into being a social work type role. I'm thinking of the guys that we work with actually, because I feel like I have more in common with them than I have with the successful people in this world, and that's the truth.

I think what I admire in people, and like to think that I have, is courage. I think when you're talking about mental illness, it's the courage that you need. That's the quality of being able to front up to it in some way. I can relate that very much to people who have psychoses of various kinds because their courage is a daily grind, it's getting out of bed, it's bothering to wipe their arse, you know. I'm their advocate. That's why I am in this game. I advocate for these people in a mental health system which actually discriminates against them, and speaks *for* them and *at* them, but which doesn't listen to them. And I'll have on the lot over that, from the Minister down, because these guys are ignored.

At the moment I feel I've been given an opportunity to actually get it right. Not in that old right/wrong sense but *actually* get it right.

Tessa Thompson

Tessa is thirty-one and works as the anti-discrimination team leader and analyst at the Mental Health Commission.

The first time I had a doctor talk to me about it was at university when I was eighteen. I went to the doctor about something else, and he suggested I go to the counsellor. The counsellor told me I had to go to the psychiatrist at Student Health. The psychiatrist told me that I was suffering from depression and I needed to take certain drugs. All this happened in very quick succession. It was shocking for me, as I wasn't expecting it.

I didn't tell anyone at that point.

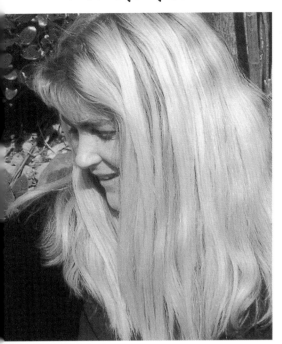

Photograph by Julie Leibrich

8 months pregnant with twins, at Pukerua on my twenty-first birthday.

But I learnt a bit about the medical model of depression.[1] So that was the first time that I thought, *Okay, I'm suffering from depression.* I certainly didn't think at that point that I had a mental illness, I just thought I had been through a rough patch. After that, it was really bad a number of times, but I managed to get back up again.

About eight years later I hit rock bottom. I wanted to die. I didn't want to carry on, and I couldn't carry on. I was like a heap. It was the week that my grandmother died. In the morning, I couldn't get out of bed. I couldn't send the kids to school. I couldn't do anything, just literally couldn't do anything. I don't know what actually happened. Somebody must have rung somebody as my children were looked after and I ended up in the doctor's waiting room.

The doctor wanted to admit me to hospital. I wondered what the hospital would offer me – an excuse to rest, an excuse I could give to other people, to tell them that I had to stop. So that's what I did – stop. Due to other support, I managed not to go into hospital, but went somewhere where I was able to go to bed for a week.

I think I've been learning how to recover ever since that rock bottom point. Of course, there have still been very bad times, up and down, and I have had a variety of different drugs and counselling since then. Sometimes I feel, *Here I am again. Why am I not in control?* I think to myself *Here I am again.*

Every time you think you're getting it right, you punish yourself severely if you get to that bad place again. One of my recovery messages for myself is that if you do get there again, you mustn't punish yourself for that. That just makes it worse. There are no good things about being there, but it's a real thing, and it's me. It's part of who I am.

The pills I took, when I first saw a psychiatrist, took me 'out'. It was as if all of a sudden my life was on television. The drugs stopped me feeling emotionally involved in my life, but they also stopped me feeling trapped, so that was great.

I was enjoying myself in a sense

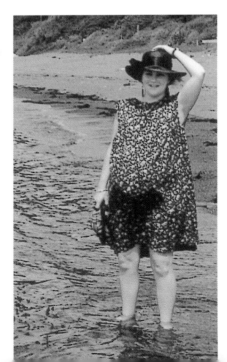

but I was watching it on TV, and it was a soap opera. All this drama was going on and I was just a thing watching it. It wasn't until I had a fight with a boyfriend that it suddenly dawned on me. *Bloody hell! I'm not emotionally involved in this. Three months ago, this would have been very powerful for me.* That was a shock, so I stopped taking the antidepressants.

I didn't think drugs were a good idea at that point, because of that emotional detachment. I suddenly felt responsible for really hurting some people in my life. I suppose it was a kind of self-realisation period as well. At eighteen, you are starting to realise how your actions impact on other people. So I didn't take drugs for a long time.

These words, which I wrote at that time, show where I *was* back then, and show me how far I've *come*. I was in a river, but in the rapids. Now I am in control, and I am swimming.

Zen in the Art of Depression 1986

flow rigid like jagged water, along a 'way',
a mugged reality moving on spontaneity
outside, not me, trip me up, let go, take me out,
should be freedom, but is lost,
kidnapped, obscured from my own
not big, no gold, not bright and purple but subtle, black, not bold
am I imploring? muzzled, mugged, muted, mutated, neurotransmuted,
neurotransmitted revelation littered
a haemorrhaging 'way', an energised casualness
unwept utterances, unkept, unkempt, all incapable, disorganisational
hassled, wasted purposeless sleepless hype, a disintegration
please don't follow me,
no enlightenment here, connections displaced. Forgotten events before they
happen,
mistakes
repeated
my independence without me involved
they're coming, they're taking, me out

Now, I have a number of ways that I handle the feeling that I'm in the rapids. First of all, I don't look for other people to try and solve it, because that only makes things worse. You can't actually tell someone that's how you feel, because then they will react. And you don't want that. You don't want to put that shit onto somebody else.

One of things I do is something I call visualisation. You can visualise an escape or any kind of story and see where that gets you. You go off into your own world and take yourself on a virtual journey. The important thing is that you take yourself all the way through the visualisation to a resolution point. The starting point might be something big – you might win a whole lot of money, maybe everyone dies (that's a kind of worst-case scenario!) or it could just be that you move to Sydney and don't know anybody.

The thing is that as I become immersed in a fantasy, it becomes like reality and I find myself unsatisfied. 'The escape', whatever it is, doesn't

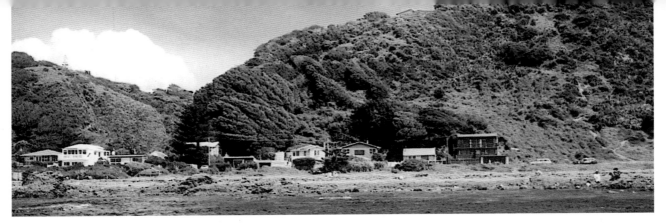

Pukerua, my ancestral home.

work. Visualisation helps me discover and rediscover that drastic action isn't necessary to escape from myself, and what I really need only requires a small action. It might be that all you need to do is be by yourself in the bush. I discover that I don't need to build a new train or blow it up. I just have to get one small wheel back on the tracks and she'll be right.

It's that simple. Somehow, in your mind, you've got in such a tangle that you just can't bear to be in it. Your imagination helps you untangle yourself.

Maybe it's a cathartic project, it allows you to shift things around in your life, experimentally, without the dire consequences of real life change. In some respects it makes you feel better about where you are right now. Or it puts it in a picture you can deal with. It removes you *slightly*, shifts you from where you are.

Another revelation in dealing with depression has been that other people have been there, too. And, what's more, some of them are the most wonderful and sensitive people I know. It's painful, but there is something you gain out of the experience of depression. Maybe it's like blind people can hear so much better. There is something about the tendency towards depression that gives you access to a sensitivity.

I can think and feel intuitively about everything around me. I'm passionate about things. I can get very loose, but I can get very, very tense. I can get really angry, and I can really care. But I think maybe the main thing is that I feel more in touch with what others are feeling. So I can see more of where other people are coming from and be supportive. You also have to realise what you can't do. You just have to let go. There's a lot of letting go. I can't deal with or feel everybody else's problems.

One of the other recovery things that has been helpful (maybe it's not so helpful when you're absolutely at rock bottom, but it's helpful on your way down) is enjoying those little things in life like custard tarts. I have to remind myself every now and then. It's when you're standing and looking at a view, or in the bush, or having coffee, or that custard tart. Enjoying those senses – taste, smell, sight, music. Of course you *enjoy* them, but I have learnt that you have to consciously *savour* them.

Going out to dinner. Listening to music, CDs or going to a concert. Sometimes watching programmes on TV. Having that time out and think-ing *I'm going to watch that*, and ignoring everyone saying, *Why do you watch that rubbish?* Actually doing it, doing it for yourself. You have to make the time to savour things. You have to look forward to them, plan them, do them. They're cheap and they make the world of difference. They're more important than just about anything else. And you can do them with peo-ple! I mean, these things are really special. That was a very important realisation. I didn't know other people did them all the time, anyway. I didn't know that. I always felt guilty if I ever purposely treated myself. It seemed trivial, or not real or something.

I think savouring things protects me. It gives me faith when I'm stressed in the head. It moves the space out a bit. Allowing yourself to enjoy some-thing is a very powerful thing. It's a message to yourself, that you're worth it. That life is good, and that you *are capable* of enjoying things.

When I feel depressed I sometimes hear that I've gotta be nice to my-self and say nice things to myself and gotta blah, blah, blah. And when I'm depressed, it just doesn't ring true. I had a therapist who said, *Say nice things to yourself.* I said nice things to myself, verbally for her, but quietly inside, I said *what a load of crap!* I didn't want to hear it. I did not want to hear it, because it hurt.

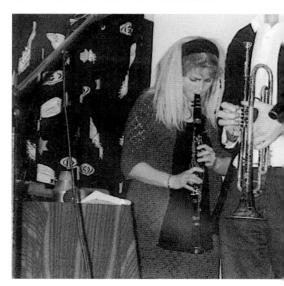

Performing 'live' at Bodega.

If I loved myself or if I accepted good things about myself, then some-thing calamitous was going to happen. And I couldn't take that chance. I would listen to the rational arguments, but the thing inside was intuitive, so you couldn't attack it through rational arguments. That's why I'm very aware that these simple things I've talked about don't sound convincing to anybody who's feeling this huge big *rrarr* inside.

I have a history of investigation in my recovery. Trying to record what I thought the problem was, looking for reasons, as well as solutions. One thing I used to do was blame. I'd blame my boyfriend or whoever was around me – 'it's because he doesn't tell me he loves me enough' or some-thing. Then after the psychiatrist told me about neurotransmissions, it was *their* fault. Then I decided it was the contraceptive pill's fault. It was all because of hormones. At one point, I thought it was a post-natal depres-sion. Then I decided it might have been because of things that happened

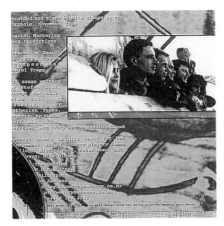

CD cover which I designed.
Great friends and good music
have been an important part
of my life.

a long, long time ago when I was a kid. There was an event that happened when I was nine years old on the beach, and it did have a very profound effect on me. So I thought it was *that* for a while. Then I looked at some other men in my life, and thought it's all *their* fault.

Now I'm way past all that blaming. It might be a mixture of all those things or it might be none of those things. It doesn't really matter. All of those things had an impact on who I am and what my life is. The blaming thing is not helpful. It's not why I am depressed that matters, it's how I deal with it.

You have to address each 'blame thing' in its own way. For brain stuff, you take drugs. For hormone stuff, for a start, you avoid the contraceptive pill. For that thing that happened when I was nine years old, I have had to go through counselling.

From some things, you'll never recover in a final sense. You go to all that counselling, get sorted out and then you get depressed again. You think, *Fuck, how come I'm depressed again?* Then your partner says, *Well, I thought you sorted all that out,* and you feel guilty. But you've got to not feel guilty, you've got to go on.

When I started work at the Commission, and I read about recovery, it occurred to me that it's an ongoing thing and I'm going to be depressed again and again and again. So that's exactly why I think this book you're interviewing me for is so special, because it's important for people to realise that it's okay to feel depressed again.

Sometimes I might ask for help. It's a huge step on my part. I don't expect people to make me feel better, but I can ask for some contact, like *Give me a cuddle.* Or, *Can I come up and have a cup of tea?* Being able to do that is important. And it's not easy.

And I have a cat. Well, it's a cuddle thing, isn't it? You can just stroke her, and she turns up when you're feeling bad. She's always there for me when I need her. Just turns up out of the blue. I don't know how or why, but she purrs.

There *is* something I think I've fixed in a final way. I experienced a huge amount of paralysis, fear and anxiety. I used to lie in bed unable to sleep, unable to move, because I was scared something would get me. I was really scared of being alone. I was scared of all sorts of situations. It was paralysing.

But I feel I've fixed that through a variety of ways. I got aropax and counselling, and particularly hypnotherapy. I know I might get depressed again but I don't think I will ever feel that terror again. Now I have myself as an adult with me as a child. Like, at Raumati Beach, I have me as an adult standing next to me as a child comforting, looking after, and preventing the fear. I hadn't realised before that even though the fear might be about something *today*, the emotion and the paralysis come from *then* – from this thing which happened to me as a child. It's a child's emotion, that kind of total fear. And you need someone to look after you.

It's so simple. All I needed to do was have me as an adult. I have complete control over me as an adult, so I can put myself with that child at any time I want, anywhere I am, at any stage. It's completely in my control and effective. To have that under control is just superb.

I don't believe I have experienced the outrageous discrimination that I know occurs, because I have avoided the hospital system, and I think that makes a huge difference in the eyes of others. It basically means I can keep it secret more easily. But that in itself is a kind of discrimination. I don't use the truth, my mental health, as an explanation for why I've been missing for a while, or what's been wrong. You can say 'I had a cold', but you can't say 'I've been depressed': not for band practice, not for a party, not for your university studies, not for your family, not for your partner, not for your job, not for anywhere.

If you do explain, some people, even close people, judge. They either think you are over dramatising, tell you not to take pills, tell you to manage your time and lose some weight and you'll be fine, or they are shocked and behave as though it changes who you are and who you have always been. Worse still, some people then start to interpret all sorts of things as 'symptoms'. So, if I am a bit angry or excited, rather than them believing that something has caused it, I have had people suggest I need to seek help from 'one of those psychobabble people I'm into'.

For the last few years I have been helped by a great GP. He seems to know what he can do and what he can't. I find him honest and sort of naïve, as he takes everything at face value. I feel like I have power because I can say anything I want and he will apply his simplistic formula. And that's all he can do, and all I can expect him to do. I'm sure he understands depression, but he doesn't know my life. He's aware of that, so he's not arrogant and he doesn't take it on board.

I don't need other people to take it on board because that's not actually going to help me. And it's certainly not going to help them. I just need people to accept it as a reality of my life. That's who I am.

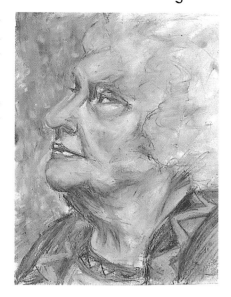

My grandmother was a painter and my inspiration.

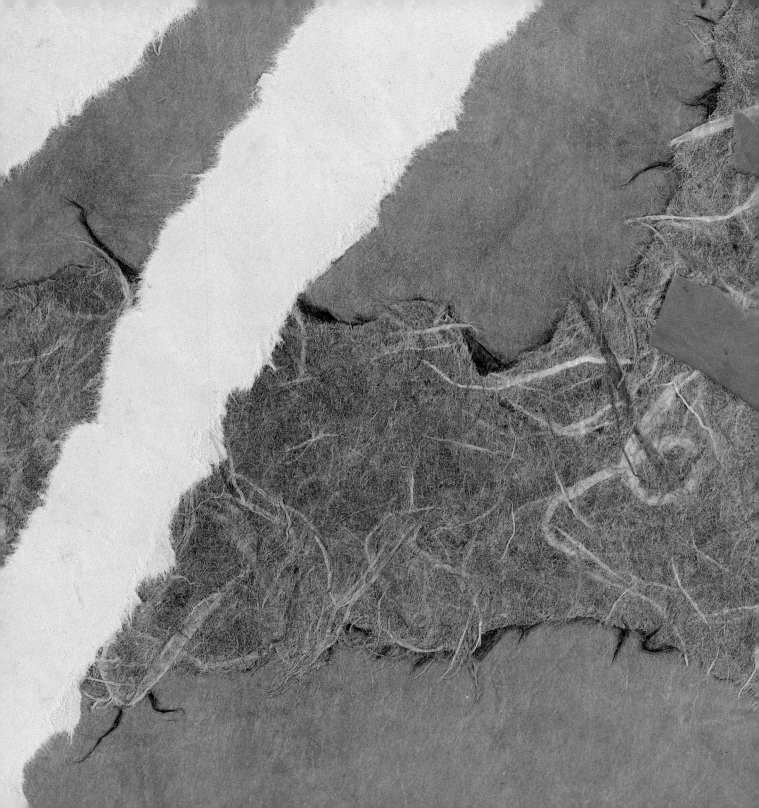

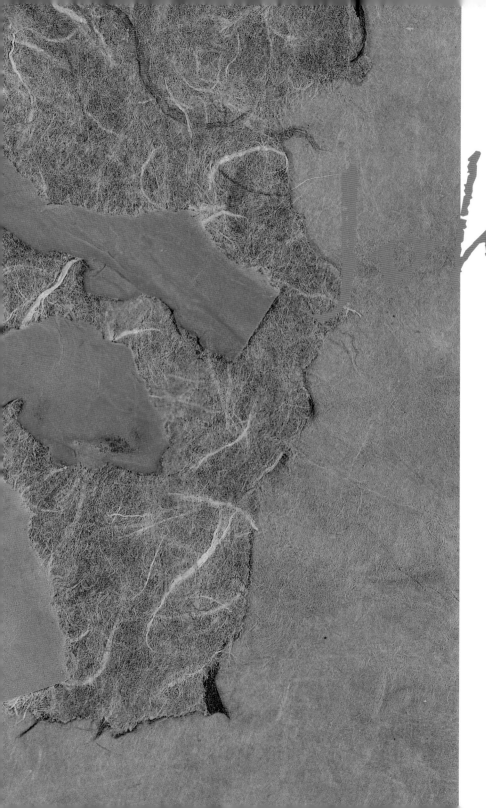

Other people share
these experiences, says

**John is a senior science stu-
dent at Otago University. His
interests include the outdoors,
pets and chess.**

I've chosen to be anonymous in this
book because I just feel that the
progress I'm making now is going to
lead to me having some sort of position of importance. And I don't want
to find, fifteen years down the track,
if society hasn't changed its perspective much, that somebody comes
knocking on my door and says, *Hey
look, we just found this book with a picture of you and a story. And gee, we didn't
know you had a mental illness, and gosh
…* you know, that could be used as a
leverage against me.

Despite there being a fair proportion of the public who are what you could term 'open-minded' and who do not view people with mental illness negatively, there are a lot who do.

I don't think anyone's really comfortable with the term 'mental illness'. It's kind of a label and I dislike labels intensely. I mean, if you're termed as having a mental illness, it sort of sets you apart from the rest of society. In fact, there are a lot of people in 'normal society' that probably walk round every day with a certain degree of mental illness. Yet they would never associate themselves with those of us who have been hospitalised at some stage.

I've only been hospitalised twice and in total for less than three months. In fact up until the age of twenty-eight I was never diagnosed with any kind of mental illness. It is a comparatively recent thing and when it did happen it was quite devastating to learn that that's how people viewed me. Basically, I had a nervous breakdown, but it's like I was given a lifetime classification. This is a difficulty I find with the system.

The worst experience I had was the breakdown itself. I became very distrustful of people. I believed that people were conspiring against me, which was a fallacy. It was a pretty frightening experience really.

It comes a lot from my background, and I guess I had a very violent, spartan type of childhood. That meant that even with my parents I had been a little bit distrustful, because there wasn't fair play at home and I knew that I could be hurt for any reason. It didn't have to be something to do with me, just the fact that I was there.

So in my late teens I found that very, very difficult and I carried a lot of hate round with me. It exposed itself a lot of the time, but I pushed it as far into the back of me as I could. When I left school (which was in the early eighties) I found it hard to get a job. The other thing I found was that because of my background I was also sort of excluded from 'the club'. When I applied for public service jobs and things like that I'd always come in close but I was never quite one of them.

I know I carried around a lot of baggage with me and it made me a very unattractive prospect for relationships with other people. So despite doing extremely well in the studying aspect, my social life was really bad.

I would say I probably had the first tremor when I went back-packing up north, shortly after finishing the first year of my qualification. I virtually had a breakdown. I just wanted to throw everything away. I found life to be pretty hard and cold, and I really was carrying a lot of baggage. And, as I learnt when I back-packed, if you carry too much weight you can't go very far.

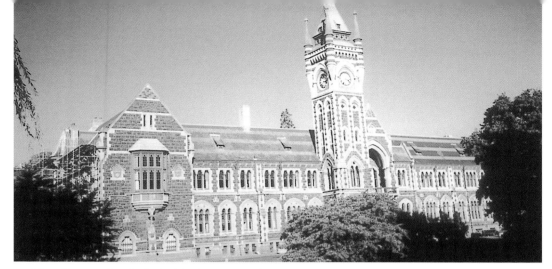

After I came back, I decided to get rid of some of that weight, so I thought about seeing a psychologist to try and remedy some of these problems that were left over from my childhood. I decided that the first thing that I had to do, despite my past, was to rectify things with my family, which I did. I spent a bit of time with my parents – didn't stay in their home but I liaised with them and tried to pick up some of the strings that were broken. This worked.

When I came back to some of the friends that I had here, I found that things had cooled off rather. So it wasn't long before I went back up north again. Anyway, by this time I decided that I'd like to travel. I think it was a form of escapism. I also felt I hadn't been prepared as a child to really have fun, to really enjoy myself, and I wanted to go somewhere.

I viewed Australia as an option, so I worked in Perth. I did find a certain amount of warmth, an openness among the Australians. But despite the regular contact, it was a very lonely time. Socially I didn't know anyone in depth, so I left my job and travelled up north to the Pilbara, where I tutored a group of young Aboriginal school children. I found an openness about them that allowed me to enjoy my time with them.

When my teaching contract expired, I was enthusiastic to get back into studying in Perth. I could no longer afford to stay in comfortable accommodation and lived in a sort of crummy apartment building, and I didn't know any of the neighbours. I got very lonely. I just lived basically to study, and as things ended up, I got paranoid.

What was happening was that I heard these sounds. First of all, it started with the person above me who had all these kids, and it was a wooden floor, and they used to run round and make lots and lots and lots of noise. My flatmate left the apartment because he couldn't stand the noise. Alone,

I used to get so frustrated. I would go up and ask them, *Please, please, please would you keep your kids from jumping up and down on the floor?* They said fine, but they never did anything. It just kept happening and happening, and frustrating me more and more. And I had to stay up later and later to actually do some work.

They moved out and that was great. I thought, *Here's a chance, maybe they'll just get a nice couple in or a single person or something,* but I guess by that stage I was starting to get quite unwell. When they were gone, I still heard these sounds. It's like it just continued. This is when I realised something must be wrong.

I realised that I was getting paranoid so I went along to the hospital and asked them if I could see a psychiatrist. No, they said that I had to see a GP first. So I went and told a doctor about it. She said *Oh, they must have kids up there. Look, if you've got all this frustration, how about we give you some happy pills to boost you up.* So I had these happy pills and that just blew me out of the ceiling. I'm not sure what they were called. They were just little tablets. After I took them, they would make me feel really, really good. Artificially really good. I couldn't help smiling. But they also further distorted my perception of what was happening around me. So in the end, I just gave up.

I've got to admit, though, that other people around the place had recognised that I had started to have an illness. But rather than knocking on my door and saying, *Hey, look, come and sit down, let's talk about it,* they tried to get rid of me because they didn't want me around.

I decided that I must shift flats. So I went out to this other set of flats, recommended to me by the landlord. There were only four flats in this block, which was good, and the top flat was available so I figured this would be ideal. I spoke to the lady there. She said, *Great, not a problem, but before you sign your contract you're going to have to sign one that will release you from where you are now.* I thought that was a bit … Anyway, I went and signed it and then I went back to her. The door was closed, the blinds were down. I knocked. No answer. So I waited for a couple of hours, knocked again, and I heard this voice from inside the office saying, *Go away.*

So I came back to New Zealand and stayed with my parents. During the time I'd been in Australia I'd rung them up regularly just to try and build bridges, and when I came back they were reasonably supportive. But then my father said, *You've to get a job and move out of here as soon as you can.* So I went to stay with my Nan. I was really plummeting by this stage; I was getting really depressed.

But one day my father did what he had done when I was very young, which was he tried to beat me. But I beat him up. I didn't break any bones but I felt like running his head through a window, I hated him so much. My mother stepped in as she had done when I was a kid once. When I was a kid my father once beat me up in the hall and my mother came over and I thought, *Gosh, she's going to stop it.* All she actually did was – she took the glasses off my face. I always felt a lot of hate towards my mother after that – the fact that she hadn't cared about me, just that it would have cost her money if the glasses had got broken. So I threw a punch at my mother when she tried to intervene.

After that my Nan came over to me and asked me to stop, so I stopped. But by this time someone had contacted the hospital. Two policemen and a psychiatric nurse arrived at the door and said, *Well, perhaps you'd like to come down and talk it over.* There was no talk of committal or anything like that, but I knew that they would commit me if I didn't agree, so I just said,

With Aboriginal school children in the Pilbara Region of Western Australia.

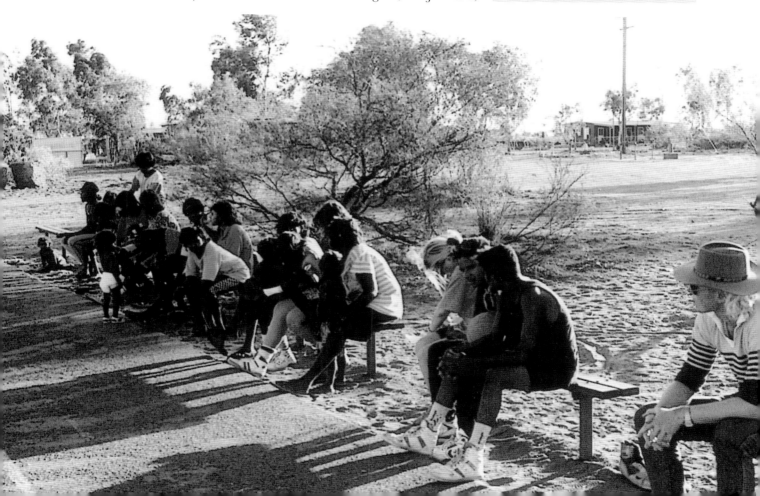

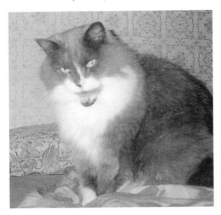

Sweetie-Pie.

Okay, fine. I was quite happy to get out of that situation, anyway.

So then I had about two-and-a-half months in hospital, during which time I was quite angry. I kept it within, and I was discharged into a PACT hostel.[1]

From my own perspective I saw myself as having had a nervous breakdown. A major one. I was not violent. I was not having a high, like a manic-depressive. I guess I was hearing sounds. I never told them that. I just simply told them what had happened and the doctor there gave me the label 'schizophrenic'. Bad news label. Since then I've learnt it's the first label that they give most people in the system.

I remember Jonathan Miller on a programme called *Madness*, on a series on the BBC television. He said the psychiatry profession woke up one morning to see two peaks on the horizon, one was schizophrenia, one was manic depression. You're either one or the other.

It's a label that I've carried ever since. One of the problems was that they gave me an antipsychotic called chlopromozine, which most people get when they go in. Then I went on to stelazine, and then they transferred me over to Piportil – pipothiazine palmitate, which is a depo injection, which I know that they'll keep me on.

After they discharged me, I went into a Level III hostel.[2] It was very nice but I was quite scared really. There were some fairly chronically unwell people there. On the other hand, there were people in the same situation as me, which was good because it gave me a chance to sit down with them and share ideas. For the first time, I guess, I shared a little bit of background with people and felt confident about doing it.

I think that place taught me a lot. It taught me how to make friends. (It's something that I had done in a haphazard way prior to going there, but I hadn't any confidence.) At the hostel I started to realise that, *Hey, other people do share these experiences!* And although I've got to admit that the prognosis for most of the people there wasn't that good, at least it gave me a chance to feel like I was at home. There was no one there saying, *Hey, you've to get out.* It's like it almost repeats in my mind, *Hey, you have got to get out.* It happened in Australia. People wanted me out, people didn't want me around. It happened at my parents'.

It was good because Paul, the manager there, said, *There's no time limit on this, just settle back and we'll work you through a routine, get you a key worker whom you can relate to and share anything you're feeling, and once a month we'll sit down and we'll talk about what sort of direction you want to go in.* In some ways it was quite lazy because everything was virtually done for you, but it was good. I really enjoyed it and got a lot out of it.

I was there the best part of two years. There was a total change within me. A total change. I remember the person who started it off. It was Merl, one of the clients there, who was a true 'Southern Woman' type of lady. Rough, not coarse – but she would get round like she was in the country, and she was always using her booming voice, and she would always poke you in the ribs and tell you to give a response. She wanted a response, she would never accept someone ignoring her, so that was good. She got me to be more outward.

She had a really positive effect on me. She got me to do a lot more laughing and joking. I was so inward and vulnerable, and she sort of changed me so that I never feared expressing myself or making jokes. *Don't even care if anyone laughs or not, just make them anyway* … Yeah, real go-getter type of person.

The hostel is also where I met my wife, which is really neat. She entranced me. I thought she was an amazing person, and we related so well, we could laugh together so well. We didn't have any fear of sharing things with each other. We used to go for walks in the park and go for coffee. Little coffee shops and cafés and things like that.

We gradually built up a relationship of real trust, and the one quality that she said she liked in me the most was my gentleness, which is really good. I mean, I never really latched onto the male macho thing. I thought that was rubbish. So it was really good to find someone whom I could share with.

Postscript

Since our interview, my wife and I have grown more in love with each other. We both feel very settled, we have been in our cottage for three-and-a-half years now – and we have a cat called Sweetie-Pie! My university studies have been going really well. A lot of people at the university know of my disability and they are very supportive. Now, I'm happy.

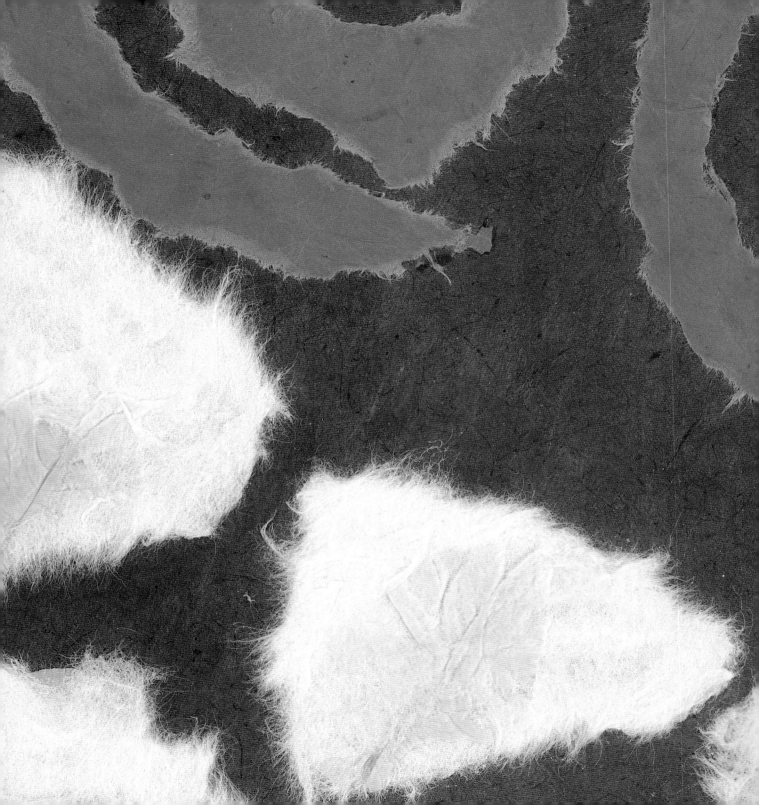

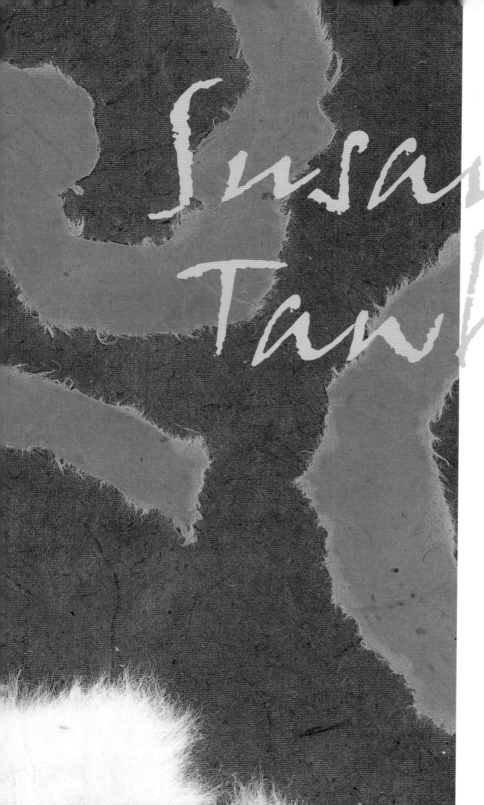

Now the time is right,
says

Susan Tanhai

**Susan is forty-five, mother of
two, grandmother of four. She
works as a service co-ordinator
for Tuia Maori mental health
services at Middlemore Hospital.**

I don't like being defined as being
mentally ill because I'm proud of the
fact that I'm mentally well and have
been so for fifteen years. Perhaps I
haven't been ill for fifteen years but
it doesn't mean to say that I haven't
been slightly unwell from time to
time.

My story's pretty basic. My experiences of unwellness started from
post-natal depression and I lived in
a big black hole for about two or

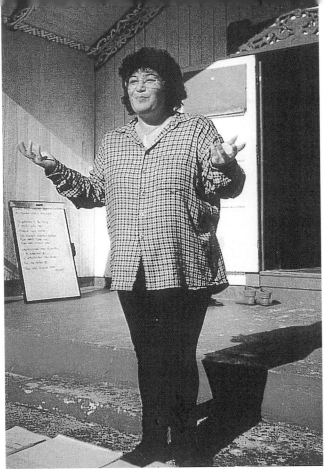

Speaking at the Potaka Marae on the East Cape.

three years. Nobody knew I was doing that because I'm really quite good at covering up things that are going on inside me. And so for those two or three years nobody knew. They just thought I was 'normal' – I made sure I looked 'normal'.

I was really careful about where I went and what I did and who I did it with. My mother didn't know and my husband didn't care, and anyway I didn't care that he didn't care. It didn't matter. I think maybe it had an effect on my daughter, who was a baby at the time.

Since then I've had two quite bad episodes of psychosis and one time where I just completely broke down, physically and mentally.[1] I knew something had happened to me but I didn't want anyone to know and although I went into a psychiatric ward, luckily it was in a general hospital. They treated what happened to me as a physical illness.

Even though I came out of hospital medicated to the eyeballs with antidepressants and quite severe psychotic medication, the whole process didn't identify as being mentally unwell. So again I was able to hide the fact from everyone that it had happened to me. The antidepressants helped me to look as though I was functioning, although I don't remember functioning. I don't remember a lot of two or three years after that because of the medication.

It's only been very recently that I have been able to look up the drugs that I was on, and see what they actually do to people. They're still on the commonly prescribed list and the drug companies say they're not addictive. But it also says that they shouldn't be prescribed for longer than three months. And I took them for three years.

I have yet to take the step of going back and saying *Why? Why did they give those drugs to me back then when they knew that this was going to happen? Why didn't they tell me I'd had a nervous breakdown?* I didn't know what was happening to me. It was really frightening, but they didn't say what I could expect to happen. Of course, they didn't tell me because it hadn't happened to them.

So that had a huge impact on my life. Over a three-year period it was quite destructive to my short-term memory. So now I have to write people's names down before I talk to them. I can't remember telephone numbers and I have to write down little notes as I'm talking to people. It's a common symptom of the medication. It's not a side-effect. It's a *symptom* of medication use. The best time was coming off the medication – that was the best time for me.

I consider myself to be fully recovered. Recovery for me is being able to look at what has happened to me in my life, face it and then deal with it. Recovery to me isn't getting rid of the symptoms of the illness.

There are certain safeguards that I've put in place and I've been able to face some of the faults I thought I had and deal with them. For example, not taking ownership of other people's problems. Just being able to address my problems, tells me that I have made a full recovery.

I think personal relationships are a really important thing, for me. It's been the ending of personal relationships that have made me crumble. I've been married twice and both were disasters. I look back and think, *Perhaps I just shouldn't be married, this doesn't suit me, it's not healthy for me to be in a relationship where someone may have some power over my decision-making.*

We parted company because I realised that living in that situation wasn't healthy for me. I've had little bouts of unwellness – panic attacks, anxiety attacks, slight depression – whenever I get into that sort of relationship. So I've learnt that I can't be part of a relationship like that. It's not that I wouldn't *like* to be in a marriage-type relationship, it's just that it's not healthy for me.

One safeguard in respect of relationships is to make it absolutely impossible for me to have one that is going harm me. I have decided that I'm not good marriage material. I like relationships up to a point and then I don't allow myself to go past that point because it's not good for me and my health.

I become emotionally dependent on people very easily. Now that's fine if it's family members like my children. To a certain extent I guess I am emotionally dependent on them because they have been protective without being overpowering since they were little kids. They understand me because they know me so well. So I can afford to be emotionally dependent on them. But not on someone that I don't know and who doesn't know me.

I didn't want my children to grow up feeling insecure, not being able to make decisions because I'd made them for them. I didn't want them being owned by someone else, not being able to make their own choices. It's a philosophy that I have stuck to all the way through and still do. So I have never owned my children. They grew up saying, *My mother never owned me!*

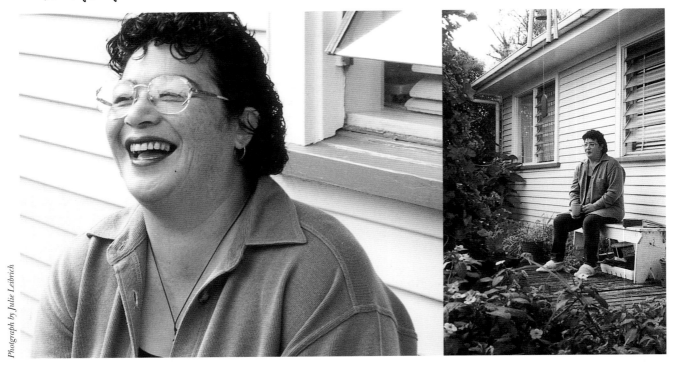

Photograph by Julie Leibrich

Outside my whare.

My own parents were really proud of me. My father was quietly proud of me and always acknowledged that he was proud of me and what I did. My mother didn't do that. She would tell other people how good I was all the time.

I have always been a very competitive person, if you like, right from when I was very small. From the age of two I played the piano and by the age of six I had my own piano. And I felt that all my life I had to perform and be competitive.

I think I expected too much of myself because of the examples my parents had set. Every time they had to pay for my music lessons I knew that they were sacrificing something else in order for me to do it, which put the pressure on me.

The other thing that really distressed me was that I had some real natural musical talent that was suppressed because of the music lessons that I took. I really enjoyed learning how to play classical music and I still like to play it, but now I listen to heavy metal! I'm really angry because the natural creativity within me was shut down through the music lessons.

My piano has been my friend for too many years. Mum said that when I was young and I was depressed, I'd play Beethoven, when I was happy I'd play Mozart and when I felt really really cheerful, I'd play more modern stuff or I'd try and compose something.

I don't have my piano now, but I've given it to someone who loves it and when I'm feeling like I need to play, I can go to her house and play it. I have an electronic keyboard, but of course there isn't the range to get the frustrations out.

I love my mother and I know I have to spend time with her and I know that she is going to say things that are going to upset me. I face that because of the love that I have for her. There were things that I hadn't talked to my mother about until very recently. And over the years I have learnt to say to her that I don't want her to talk about some things because of what that does to me. It is not just defence, it's building some protection around me as well.

I have all these protections that I use. If I am going somewhere, I make sure that I am not going to expose myself to something that I know is not going to be good for me, or good for my health. I like to plan things and I like things to go to plan. If they don't go to plan I go to pieces, so I have to be in control of that plan and other people just have to understand that.

Like, when I first moved to Auckland I lived in a flat with three other people. I'd left all my friends in Huntly and I'd never been flatting before. I didn't know these people and they didn't know me. I made it very clear right from the start that I couldn't be their mother, or their therapist, but would be their friend. They had to learn how to understand me, so that I was still protected. But they never ever learnt it. They knew about my depression, and if I went into my room for some time out they thought I was becoming unwell. They didn't understand that I just needed some time for me. And they would try to entertain me. Like they'd say, *Let's go out to the movies. Let's go out to dinner.* They were mistaking my aloneness, my need to be alone, for depression.

I need to be able to say to people that I need to go to my room. It's not because of you or something you've said but because it's time for me to be alone and spend some time doing things for me. You don't have to organ-

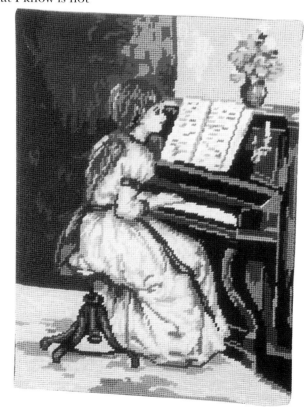

Tapestry made by my mother.

ise things for me to keep me occupied. *I know how to keep myself well and part of that is having time out on my own*. But sometimes I need to be able to say to people that I need to be with you.

At work, I like to have a cut-off point. At five o'clock I knock off and that's all there is to it. When I get phone calls at the weekend or at night, I'll say to people, *That's fine, I will ring you tomorrow at such and such a time and we will get the matter sorted out then, because there is nothing I can do right now.* That's something I learnt in time management.

I make it effective for the organisation, but there is no use me spending all my time doing one thing and burning out at the expense of all the other things that need doing as well. So I don't try and take it all on and do the whole lot. I make sure that I recognise my cut-off level, my boundaries.

Because I like to be organised, I need to tell people how I like to do things. I'm okay about sitting in the work team and saying, *I need to have a three-hour lunch break today because I need to get away from you all.* I need to be really honest about how I do my work.

I'm one of those people who can't sleep at night with the window shut in my room. I close my bedroom door and I open the window. It's like an escape route. I've always had this fear about the house burning down, ever since I was a little girl, and so I have everything in an orderly fashion in my room.

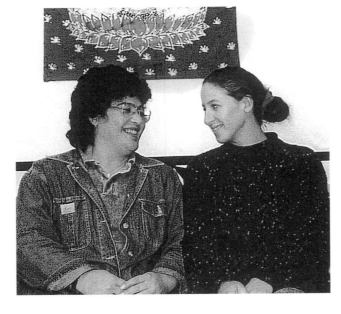

With my daughter, Denise.

When I was a little girl I prioritised the most important things in my life and I made sure that they were together so that if the house caught on fire I could grab, in order of priority, what was important to me and take it out of the house. To be closed in and not be able to escape has always been a phobia of mine, and I guess that I never sat and examined the emotional issues around that.

People delve into their emotions when they are ready to. And there are some things in my life that I am just too scared to delve into. One day I might, but I am not overly concerned about it because I don't see that has got any relevance to my staying well. I don't need to do this yet. All I need to do is make sure that I get up every morning and go to bed every night.

All of us want to know why. At the end of the day you go back to where you came from to find out why. In the early days, Maori lived at home in their whanau situation. If you started to hear voices or you were showing signs that you weren't the same as everyone else, you were accepted as being like that. You could be considered to be gifted, and so there was an answer for you straightaway because you were right there and there were people that could tell you why. Now, it's different.

I had no links with my ancestors or with where I came from. And I had no links with the people who could tell me why I am like I am. My belief is that if I had known who I was and known myself better I would have been able to cope better with the depression.

For a long time my priority was to find those things out because I was unwell too often and I thought that that was why. And I kept getting told that when the time is right I will find those things out. But because I'm an organised person, I thought that I needed to know those things in my head, because I couldn't understand the things that were in my heart.

And so I became obsessed with having to find out why I was like I was – while on the other hand being really terrified about having to make that journey. And so what I had to do was listen really carefully to what the old people were saying. And that was *When the time is right it will happen.* No one was saying to me, *Okay, let's get this out of the way now so it's not a problem for you any more. I* was making the problem. I had all these feelings of inadequacy because I am obviously a Maori woman. People can see I am a Maori woman. I wanted to be able to show them I'm a Maori woman, how Maori I was, and I thought I had to tell them who I was.

I don't have te reo, and I always felt discriminated against because of that. Non-Maori society sort of expects that you can speak Maori and that you should understand it. And more than anything I had to be accepted as a Maori but I didn't want anyone again to know that I had all these inadequacies inside me. Which is why I became obsessed with having to find out who I was.

So now, I've listened to what people said and I've put the obsession onto the back-burner. I really, really want to be able to tell my grandchildren about their ancestors. About where they're from and to give them a sense of belonging to their people.

And so now the time is right and I'm ready to go on the journey.

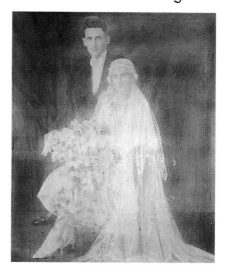

My grandparents.

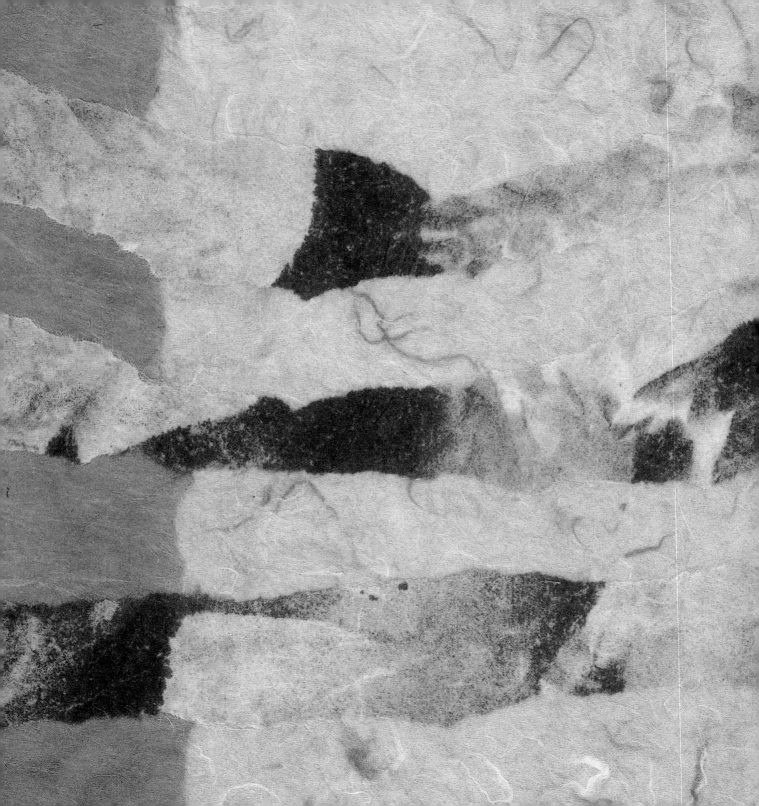

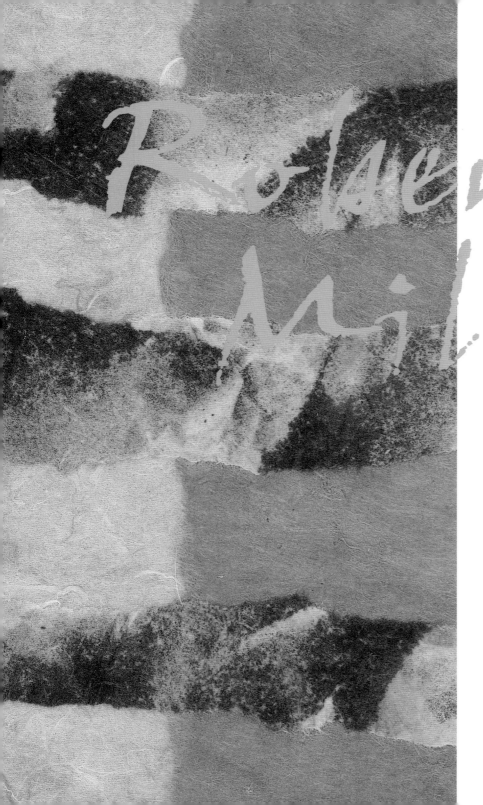

Learn the maximum
amount, says

Robert Miller

**Robert is Associate Professor
in the Department of Anatomy
and Structural Biology at
Otago University. He has spent
many years researching brain
function including disorders of
the brain in schizophrenia. He
is fifty-five, likes tramping and
a wide range of music.**

As an adolescent at school I guess I
was not thriving, in mental health
terms, and I hadn't had many good
relationships or close friends. But I
did well enough to go to university
as a medical student and worked
hard at that, although I was also becoming progressively more and
more overwhelmed by rapid, pow-

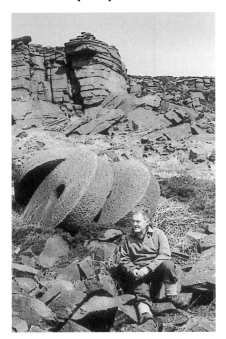

My father at Stanage Edge, South Yorkshire, which I still regard as my spiritual home ... also the origin of millstone grit, the stone used in past times to sharpen steel in the Sheffield cutlery industry. My father died in 1995.

erful fluctuations of mood. Eventually I found myself being a clinical student at one of the London teaching hospitals. At the time it was pretty grim. I mean, being a medical student in London, with no friends, trying to learn medicine, at the same time having fearfully embarrassing situations with patients, to whom I had no hope of relating; and also going down with a psychotic illness, which I didn't understand. I didn't know what was in store for me in the future. That was all pretty bad.

I was eventually overwhelmed by a psychotic breakdown in November 1967, which came on within minutes; and I was admitted to hospital in Sheffield forcibly. The following day, I absconded from hospital and went to the hills. There was a snowstorm forecast. It was a suicide bid. I wanted to finish things in the Pennine hills, which had meant a great deal to me when I was an adolescent. After that I was in hospital for six months.

After I got out of hospital I was still on neuroleptics. I know now that I was on far too large a dose – about ten times too large. I was therefore severely sedated. I was scarcely employable. I thought, *This is part of what I am now*, and I didn't know that it was really an effect of too large a dose of neuroleptics.

This went on for two or three years after the first episode; I really thought I was finished. That's a long time at the age of twenty-four. I had a few odd jobs during this time and then I landed a job as a research assistant in Glasgow. At the same time, the psychiatrist who was in charge in Sheffield said, *I think we should try tailing off the medication now.* So I tailed them off completely, and felt much better. But I started to become psychotic again, quite quickly. Soon the thoughts in my mind were so unpleasant that they made me feel ill, and because they made me feel ill, I started taking the medication again, which saved my bacon.

When I was a PhD student I was playing around with the dose of the drugs to try and work out what I really needed, and this was all done single-handedly, without any guidance, which I don't recommend. I didn't really become convinced that there was some sort of future for me until 1972, when I got a PhD. Even then it was not so straightforward because, PhD or not, if you have got a history of a serious mental illness you are not going to get a job. However, I did get a post-doctoral position and was gradually coming off the medication. Then I went on a brilliant holiday climbing mountains. In the next month nothing important was happening to put me under any psychological stress and I stopped the medication completely. But I still went psychotic.

So I had set it up in a way to learn the maximum amount. It was an experiment, it was a good one which gave a decisive conclusion, although in personal terms it was a disaster. I was admitted to hospital again. I voluntarily went to hospital that time. I was only there for two or three weeks and then psychiatrists realised I could cope outside.

There had been no discrimination against me when I got the post-doctoral position in Britain. But I had been told that I was unlikely to get an academic post at that university, so I applied for a job at another university.

After that, I was always up-front with information about my mental illness, because I thought if this really is prejudice you want to force it out into the open. I succeeded at that at one later interview. I was interviewed for a lecturer position and someone on the committee said, *What sort of illness was it that you suffered from?* So I said it was a schizophrenic illness. Well, that person actually backed me for the job, but I only got a temporary job, a six months lecturing job.

Later on (about 1976), I was offered a longer term position in New Zealand. I went to see the acting head of a department and I asked him for advice. He said, *I advise you to take the job in New Zealand: with your health record you don't stand a chance of getting a permanent academic position*. So I had forced it into the open.

When I got to New Zealand I wrote a letter which was published in the newsletter of National Schizophrenia Fellowship in Britain, documenting what had happened. In it, I asked the question: *How many medical schools in Britain, as a matter of policy, refuse to accept as members of academic staff those who have had a psychotic illness?* No one has ever answered. I would like to ask that question again.

Over the years I've certainly experienced prejudice. For instance, on one occasion, when I was giving a research talk, a fairly high-up academic, who might well have seen my CV, said in public: *Anyone who believes that must have a deranged mind*. Another example was when I went to an evening class on psychiatric topics. When I said that I myself had suffered from a psychotic illness and described myself as an ex-patient, a psychiatric nurse there raised her eyes to the ceiling and said: *Are you ever an ex-patient?*

Nowadays, there are a lot of people who come into the mental health professions with some sort of personal experience of mental illness. In their different ways, they will be drawing on those experiences. But there are some people who have been mentally ill, who find it impossible to recognise what has happened to them. And so they are unable to integrate this fact into the rest of their lives. Some of these people even build elaborate castles in the air to avoid confronting their history of mental illness.

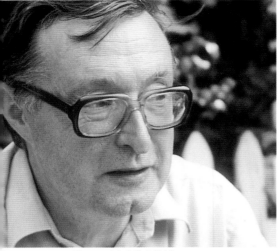
Photograph by Julie Leibrich

These castles are not psychotic delusions; they are a different sort of delusions – they're defence mechanisms.

During my first episode in hospital, no one ever mentioned a diagnosis. And I never asked. We went on like this, you know, stone-walling each other for about three years. Then the second time I was in hospital, which was just for a few weeks, one registrar, I remember the occasion, he sort of pulled himself together for what might have been a difficult session and said, *What do you think the nature of this illness is?* So I told him I thought it was a schizophrenic illness, and he said: *That's right.* And to make sure there was no messing he showed it to me written in the case notes.

A couple of years later, when I was in the process of emigrating to New Zealand, I saw the consultant in charge of this outfit. I mentioned to him the diagnosis of schizophrenia I had seen in my case notes and he *denied* it. There is no doubt in my mind that the registrar had a better understanding of what I needed than the consultant.

As far as I am concerned, I don't give much credence to the way diagnoses are made, but I think psychosis is a concept I recognise. I think for the illness I suffered from, the psychotic episodes are quite separate from the vulnerabilities that are there when you are not psychotic. I think that is probably true of what is called schizophrenia, and it is probably true of what is called bipolar disorder. I think you *can* make distinctions between bipolar disorder and schizophrenia, but I think they are not completely clear-cut, and that the classification leaves a lot to be desired.

Everyone tries to think categorically. That's one reason why some people are given several different diagnoses. The whole procedure of classification of people is very dodgy. You can classify animals and plants because they breed true, but you can't classify humans in quite the same way. Another common confusion is that we think of illness as categories – measles, mumps, scarlet fever. With disorders of the human person, they don't fall into categories. They merge into one another continuously, like different degrees of high blood pressure; they are dimensions not categories.

The first stage of recovery is getting over the psychotic episode. The text books say the medications work in two or three weeks, or perhaps a month, or something like that. But it seems to me that the actual ideas that come to your mind when you're psychotic are dissipated much more slowly than that. My experience, with fairly florid psychosis, is that the actual recovery period is much longer than that – six months, a year, in which you are still toying with the delusional ideas.

Recovery from the psychosis itself is two to twelve months in my experience. Working out the right dose of the right medication should be done in collaboration with a physician. To treat psychosis you don't need a dose that will sedate you completely. You need a dose that leaves you with an active mind but not an over-active mind.

The sort of professional help that might be needed is not so much saying, *You must take those medications*, but setting up some sort of a contract saying, *You may not believe me but these drugs will help you, so let's set up some sort of system. If you make a mistake and stop your medication and become psychotic, you will learn the maximum amount from your mistake.*

That's how I would like to see things set up. You can't expect people to believe that a medication can change the way you think, without having actually experienced it. So you need to convince yourself that you really need medications. Careful experimentation is needed over some years.

This is a book I wrote in 1995, in collaboration with the Schizophrenia Fellowship, N.Z., Inc., Otago Branch.

Let me just mention some of the other points about recovery. Obtaining employment is a very important step. Good luck is needed. In my case I had to emigrate. I could probably have got some sort of employment in Britain but it was clear that doors were closing on me. And to get a job offer, even if it was on the other side of the world, was something. Someone knew how to write a good letter to attract me here, and I'm very grateful.

Then other stages of recovery – repairing the damage that has been done by psychotic illness at a critical stage of life. I think from the age of two to twenty, one builds up a whole repertoire of behaviours which allows one to function in an adult world. Psychosis destroys a lot of that development, so you get to the age of twenty-five and you've got the maturity of someone of a much younger age. You have to spend an equivalent amount of time rebuilding those structures. It is particularly important with regard to relationships, self-assertiveness, and things like that.

I think personal relationships are one of the most difficult things about psychotic illness. The illness generally comes on in late adolescence and early adulthood, when most people are developing their capacity for relations, coming to terms with their own sexuality and things like that. To have that mixed up with a major psychological illness, something much bigger, much

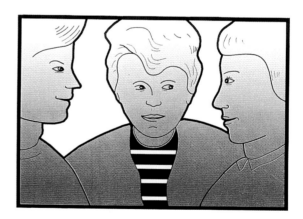

Straight Talking about Mental Illness

with emphasis on Schizophrenia

an educational guide
by
Robert Miller

Below: Manuscript from my composition **Weeping Song.**

more difficult, throws you off-course for many years to come. I think that this is something in principle that I have solved now, many years later.

Then we get on to the really long-term things. We're talking about the last ten years now. This is distinguishing between those long-term consequences of having been ill which *can* be reversed and those things which are signs of impairment and vulnerability that you are *not* going to get rid of, and you might as well learn to live with. For me, the irreversible sign of impairment is problems with attention.

I'm a university lecturer, so you might think I have pretty good powers of attention, but I hide my disabilities fairly well. In fact listening to talks, lectures, committee meetings particularly, it is absolutely amazing how little I pick up. On the other hand, if the information is coming in my preferred way, in a written form, and the information is interesting, I have great powers of concentration. Or again, when I'm asked to speak without preparation (particularly in committee meetings), I am always overwhelmed by everyone else, but when it comes to putting things in writing I do better than those people.

Sensitivity to noise – that's something that's with me for life, and the people around me at work know that I'm sensitive to noise. Sometimes when there is someone talking in the background, I can't continue a conversation with someone across the table because I hear more of the background voice than anyone else is hearing. So these are the things that I now recognise as ongoing.

It's the same thing with visual distraction as well – movements in the side of my visual field will distract me from talking or from reading. I can think of these things in neurological terms but also I know about them from first-hand experience and I know they're real.

Thinking about the very long-term recovery process, I have needed to recognise those things that I am never going to be capable of, such as enjoying parties. There was a time when I used to go to parties because everyone used to go, and you *ought* to like to go to parties. I actually hated every minute of them but I still went to them. Now I have a pretty steady life, avoiding late nights, and I guess I instinctively avoid stressful situations.

My family has been very supportive. I think my experiences of prejudice are mainly from professional people, mainly people in health services and mental health professions. That's partly because those are the people I work amongst. Of course, I choose my friends because they won't behave like that.

What has gradually got better? Self-confidence. The capacity to form close relationships. What else? Look, this thing about the strength of a personality. I think there is one sense in which someone who has a psychotic tendency has a weaker ego-strength, if you like. But there is another sense in which you could rebuild a lot of that. The experience of psychosis leads you to doubt all your own beliefs and doubt whether you can have an opinion that means anything. But that is something that you recover. You gain your confidence, in my experience, very slowly, and by very careful thought about everything you think or believe.

With the rebuilding of the psychological structures that make a personality comes your security and your beliefs. And your capacity to believe in other things gradually increases. For instance, take someone who has had religious delusions. How can they have a religious belief after that? Well, the answer is *Yes, you can.* But you have to go to a much deeper level than the things that come to you on the spur of the moment.

You never recover, in the sense that this is just one way of growing older. This is my way of maturing and facing the experiences I've had, just as everyone grows older in the face of the experiences they've had.

There are positive effects of having been psychotic; these experiences give you insight into philosophical problems that most people never come anywhere near. You are much more aware of the relationship between mind and body (or mind and brain) than most people. That is quite a profound experience over the years, and it's given me a research career in mental illness, understanding the brain mechanisms of mental illness.

Postscript

For someone who does research on mental illness, living this story has amounted to a very special education; but for a long period it was not clear that I would survive it.

About stigma and discrimination … over the last six or seven years, there has been important change. It's been slow and gradual, but quite tangible: a lifting of the burden of prejudice relating to mental illness. This looks like a vision being fulfilled. It's just the start now, but it's held worldwide by many people, community groups, university researchers, organisations like the Mental Health Commission, pharmaceutical companies, and so on. There's still a long way to go, but this change has got a lot of momentum.

To be brave
Is to behave
Bravely
When your heart is
Faint

So,
You can be really brave
Only when you really
Ain't.

I don't know where this comes from, but it is a favourite verse of mine.

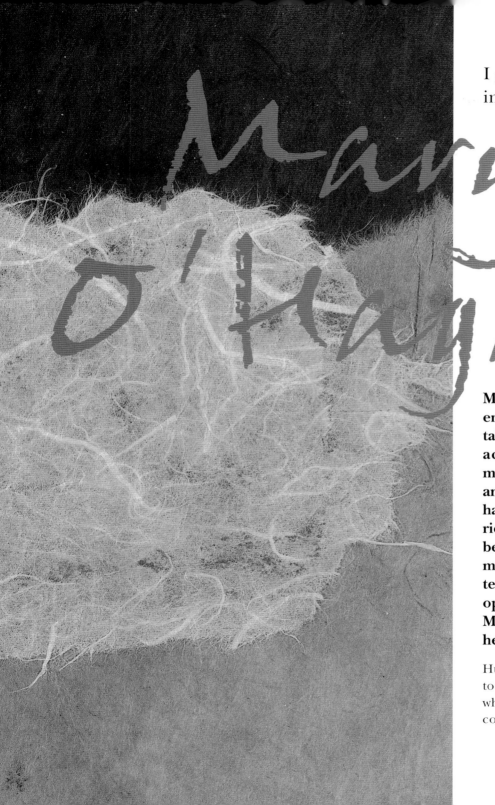

Mary O'Hagan

I gradually found a place in the world, says

Mary is forty-one and a self-employed consultant in mental health issues. She has been active in the service user movement, both nationally and internationally (and has had some interplanetary experiences as well). She is a member of the Mental Health Commission's anti-discrimination team and also works on developing the recovery approach. Mary lives in Auckland with her partner and children.

Human beings have a compulsion to find explanations for things. So what I'm telling you is my story, my construction about my life and mental illness. Because I really do think human beings make up stories. I don't think there is *a truth* out there waiting to be found. This belief comes from my experience of depression, and from my experience of coming from a family where a wide latitude of experience and belief was acceptable, and where we were encouraged to question things.

I see my mental illness as opening with the death of one of my brothers and closing with the death of another of my brothers. It's quite strange, really.

When I was ten a baby brother of mine was born. He was fine for the first couple of days, and I remember tremendous excitement. Then a phone call came and my father went away to the maternity hospital. My brother had turned blue and died several days later. That had a huge impact on me. I was old enough to be aware of the enormity of something like that, but I was too young to deal with it perhaps. I think it was the first experience I had of depression and despair.

When I read back the essays and stories I wrote during and after that time there was an awful lot of stuff going on – feelings of gloominess and isolation. I didn't have a huge depressive crisis, but as a teenager I was pretty depressed in an everyday sense, not in a psychotic sense.

My mood swings didn't get really bad until I left home at eighteen. At that age all I could see was a vast expanse of uncharted life in front of me. It terrified me. Everything seemed so uncertain. I think being young is really hard – it certainly was for me. And I think having a mental illness at that age just prolonged the angst of not knowing where my life was going.

I was in and out of hospital for eight years, until I was twenty-six. My life was just a roller-coaster really, and I couldn't do the things that other people my age were doing. It was chaos. I had very rapid mood swings, highs and lows, and the more extreme they got, the more rapid they became.

The first time I got very severely depressed I was studying theory of knowledge, which is enough to send anyone spinning. I got fixated on this old philosophical statement: *I cannot know anything for certain, not even that.* I just got steadily more depressed. I felt like I was in a black box, and that all my life, my culture, and I had colluded together to paint these lovely colourful decorations to hide the blackness. The box even had windows with views painted in them and things like that. I thought I had arrived at the terrible bare truth which was that once all the decorations were stripped away, all I was left with was blackness, you know, the deepest blackness.

Being depressed was like having a whole lot of switches turned off in my brain. I got very slowed down and withdrawn. I would also feel very vulner-

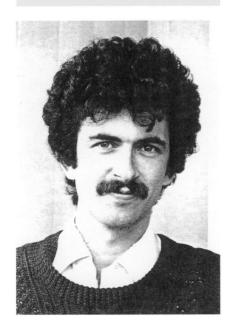

My brother Sean

able – like I had no skin. Then there were the times when I couldn't hold a thought in my head – they just got sucked into the blackness. That was scary because life is chaos without words. And all through it was my loss of hope and the terrifying belief that life was meaningless. And you know, it's an experience where there is only room for one. The isolation was pretty unbearable at times.

I got better at being depressed as time went on. I learnt to find some peace in the blackness. My whole spiritual life – not that I have a very active spiritual life – is built on the peace of blackness. I don't use light metaphors at all, although I know that is very common. But my spiritual imagery is total blackness and I find a lot of tranquillity in that.

Being high was frustrating for me because I lost my concentration very quickly and I like concentration. It was like having a great big pair of blinkers on – one blinker blocked out the past and the other blinker blocked out the future. So all I could see was the present whizzing past me – a sort of streak of speed. I just couldn't actually hold the past or future in my head. I also found that the mood was a bit tinselly as well; it wasn't very deep, I suppose, because I couldn't focus on anything. Another frustration was that it was very hard to find people who were in that state, so it was quite a lonely state to be in. The world was unbearably slow and I was really speeding.

On the whole, I didn't find the highs a very comfortable experience although there were some amazing things about them. There are pieces of music that I listened to when I was high that I listen to now, and I still have a very expansive response to them. And the colour was just incredible. When I was depressed I felt like I was walking through a sort of faded old watercolour, but when I was high the colours were just amazing.

When I was twenty-six my older brother, Sean, who was two years older than me, was drowned. I was really close to him. At that time I had just gone on an antidepressant in addition to lithium and was feeling a hell of a lot better than I had for some years. It's funny how events in life coincide sometimes.

My brother had been a successful person. He had had a few problems but he was getting on with his life. He had a great job and he had a partner and a little child. I always saw him as the lucky one. When he died I realised that he was the unlucky one, because he had been knocked off the rails at the age of twenty-eight, and I've got every chance of reaching old age. His death made me realise that self pity is a complete and utter waste of time. You've got only so long in this life, and none of us knows how long. It's so important to make the most of it. I suppose since then I've always felt quite a lucky

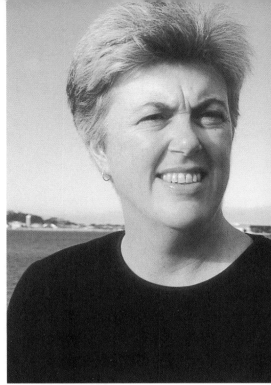

Photograph by Julie Leibrich

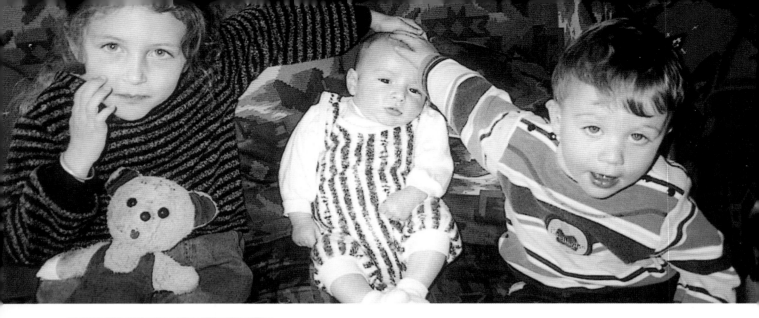

Ruby, Felix and Rupert –
my children.

person, and I think that's been helpful in my recovery.

Another way his death helped me was that my brother vacated a space which I went on to occupy. It was a kind of 'successful person' space, and although he didn't do anything to try and stop me being successful, I had lived in his shadow. Also I had this mission for a few years – I wanted to keep my brother's spirit alive and well in the world. I suppose Sean was the best friend I ever had for sharing ideas, so I wanted to continue his ideas in the world. It's like he handed me something as he was being carried down the river, and I had to go and do it.

So in a very paradoxical way, I think his death (although I wish it hadn't happened) was a bit of a launch pad for me. But if I hadn't been on the antidepressants as well it may have affected me quite differently. I'll never know.

After that time I didn't have major instability. My moods were like a ball bouncing a little less every time, and it took a few years for it to bounce out. I still take medication. I tried going off it about five years ago and ended up on the edge of that precipice thinking, *Shit, I'm going to go right down again.*

The funny thing about calling it a mood disorder is that for me it was a condition that affected every aspect of my being, not just my mood. It had just as big an impact on my physical abilities, my cognitive abilities, my sleep patterns, and my sensory experience. It seems weird just to call it a mood disorder.

My mental illness was definitely the most difficult experience I've had in my life. Well, nothing that's happened before or since has come anywhere near it – it was that hard. But I remember saying to myself when I got stable again, that if I could live through mental illness, I could live through just about anything. That's a reassuring thing to know.

When I look at the other very intense experiences people have, like being struck down by a beam of light on the road to Damascus, or falling in love, mental illness has got no positive meaning in our culture. I was left with this amazing experience but I didn't know what it all meant. They didn't help me, they just said I had a biochemical imbalance, so there was no sort of cultural container to put my experience in, that said, *This is mental illness and this is what it means.* So I was left feeling very stranded with this experience and not knowing what to do with it.

One of the things that motivated me to work in the mental health area was that I wanted to know what this thing called mental illness was all about and I wanted to know *why* it happened. And I have to say that after many, many years of considering this question, my short answer is that I don't know. I guess part of my recovery is also accepting that I can't make total sense of my experience.

I was also looking round for a job because my whole career path had been quite decimated by my years of instability. I had been at university a bit, but had to withdraw from most of my courses for medical reasons. So really, at a very pragmatic level, I was looking for an occupation and I wasn't a great prospect for most employers.

So I started off planning to write a book for people with manic depression – a kind of information and self-help book. I never wrote it, but it got me on a path. Then in 1985 I went to the Mental Health Foundation conference in Wellington. There were about 200 people there I think, and only two of them identified as having a mental illness, which I thought was extraordinary. On the last day I got up and said, *You people have been talking about people like me for two days. Why don't you ever talk to us and listen to what we have to say? It's about time you started.*

My partner Sara and me.

After that I was quite fired up and set up Psychiatric Survivors in Auckland. Then I went on to set up, with some other people, the Aotearoa Network of Psychiatric Survivors. I stayed there for two years. Later, I worked in England in a mental health consultancy for a year. Since then I have been working in New Zealand. I was the first chair of the World Federation of Psychiatric Survivors for about four years and that involved quite a lot of travel.

One thing I was very lucky about was that I didn't feel a lot of shame about having a mental illness. I think that was a huge help to me. I don't quite understand why I didn't feel shame but I always felt, you know, people ought to get medals for going through an episode of mental illness. I thought it was weird that you can go through all that hell and at the end of it you feel ashamed and other people just shun you. If you ask me, that's really adding insult to injury.

Some discrimination against people with mental illness is overt but some of it's really subtle and hard to read. I think one of the worst discriminations is internalised because it gives others permission, in a way, to discriminate against you. I found a lot of mental health professionals thought they had some sort of monopoly on insight and knowledge. That's a kind of discrimination and it used to really annoy me.

I suppose the thing that I found most discriminatory was being told at the age of twenty that I would have to lower my horizons because I had an ongoing condition. All I could see in front of me was the life of a basket weaver, impoverished, lonely, in and out of hospital. But they were so wrong. It's so daft to make predictions about anyone else's life.

I was terrified for a time that I'd never use my abilities or have a good relationship or children, because of my mental illness. If I'd known, in my moments of despair, that I was going to be as fulfilled and successful in my life as I have been, I wouldn't have believed it. It's strange how life unfolds; my fears back then turned out to be totally unfounded.

You see, in the end my mental illness opened so many doors for me. It was a terrible experience but it was also really fascinating – after all, it's quite an interesting experience to find yourself on a spaceship bound for Mars! And I've had a really interesting career because of it. And it knocked quite a few important life skills into me. That's why I hate it when mental health workers talk about the things mental illness takes away from people. I survived one of the more difficult experiences a person can have. I didn't need group therapy and social skills groups and crap like that – I just needed stability and the opportunities to accumulate some good experiences. One of the problems about having all those episodes was that I just had one bad thing happen after another. But when I became more stable I was able to start to accumulate good experiences. I think that builds on itself and life just gets better.

When I was going through all my instability, I became highly organised and tidy as a way of reassuring myself that I was well. And I remain that way to this day. It gives me an illusion of control. I mean, let's face it – being organised is not going to stop me from having a mental illness, but I think people need an illusion of control and that's my illusion. We walk around

Cover of my book, *Stopovers*.

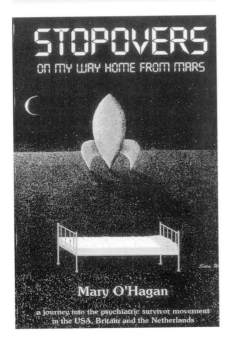

STOPOVERS
ON MY WAY HOME FROM MARS

Mary O'Hagan

a journey into the psychiatric survivor movement
in the USA, Britain and the Netherlands

in our ordinary everyday lives thinking that we are in control, but one thing I learnt from my mood-swings was what an illusion that is! I realised I couldn't will myself to stay in control. People forget 'there but for the grace of god go I' – not that I think in terms of god – you could equally say it's but for the grace of the universe, or our biochemistry, our early life experience, oxygen, water, gravity, or whatever.

I didn't lose any of my motivation between episodes, so I kept myself occupied and interested in things. And I suppose there was a bit of a fighter in there too, you know, *No bastard's gong to grind me down*, and I mean the bastards inside my head as well as the bastards out there. I think I got a lot of practice at that spirited, determined thinking as a rebellious teenager, even if I left school knowing nothing about trigonometry or grammar.

There were always people around me who believed in me, including my family. They always thought that I had been an under-performer, and that there was quite a lot in there which my mental illness hadn't taken away, just hidden. And other people opened some doors for me. People like the Mental Health Foundation who gave me office space and support to start Psychiatric Survivors, when they didn't know me from a bar of soap. That kind of thing was hugely important in my recovery. No one gets anywhere without other people opening doors for them.

I'm just really lucky that I was able to turn the experience around. I get huge satisfaction out of that. I somehow used my experience to build a life when it could have destroyed it. It's also been really important for me to be in a very happy relationship, and I've had that in recent years. Having someone who accepts you and loves you, and who you can love back, is really important. It has added the icing to the cake of my recovery. And having children has been important too.

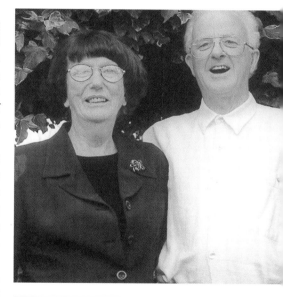

My parents.

I feel really lucky to have found a place in the world, a valued place, because my prospects didn't look too good at one stage. I was slipping into a 'chronic psychiatric patient' role, you know, one of those people the services have given up on. But I didn't give up and I gradually found a place in the world where I wanted to be. Mind you, it was hard work getting there sometimes. My life has just gradually got better and better, with just the usual ups and downs. That's what recovery has meant for me.

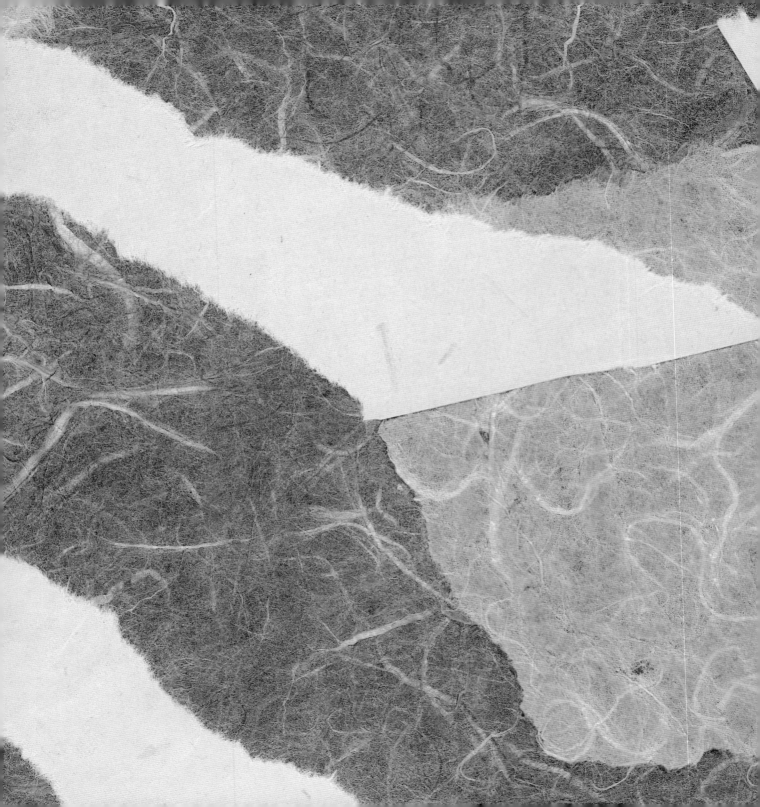

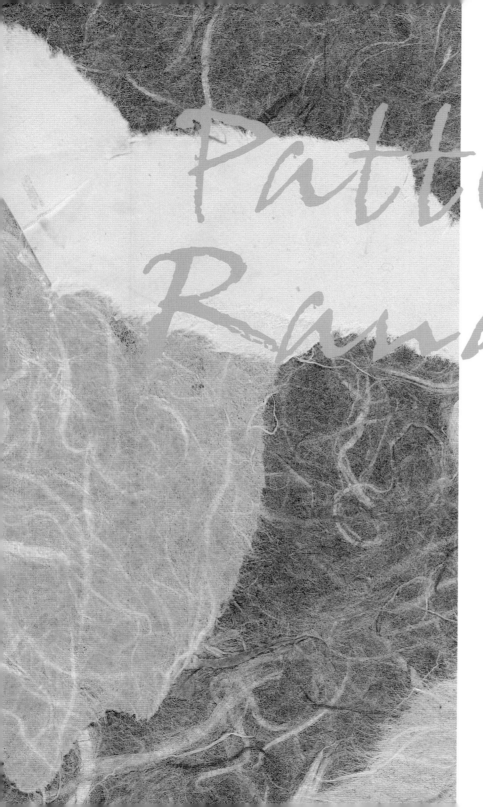

Loving relationship is at the root of recovery, says

Patte Randal

Patte is forty-seven and works as a doctor with people who suffer from psychotic illnesses. She is married and has three sons.

The first time I became unwell I was twenty-four, and that was probably triggered off by just a puff of marijuana. Literally, a puff. I think the puff really blew the whole system away.

My father had recently died, I'd had a baby, my marriage had broken up, and I was doing a PhD looking at the Chinese philosophy of health, which totally challenged my world view. All the structures that had held me in place were shaken. It sent me into an altered state of consciousness, which I think then led to my being unwell. But at the time I had no idea at all that this was psychosis.

I experienced it as a mystical experience. It was almost orgasmic in its impact on me. I experienced some kind of cosmic battle between trust and fear, between a sort of intensity of terror, and an equal and opposite intensity of some kind of joy – something extraordinarily wonderful.

The wonderfulness was what won out, was what I was left with. This extraordinary feeling, knowing that life had purpose and meaning, and that *my* life had purpose and meaning. It changed my life.

My behaviour, during that time, was obviously a little disturbed, and my friends were a bit worried about me, but basically I didn't get a diagnosis put on me, although I had very brief treatment with medication.

I was admitted to the university sick-bay and they took care of me extremely well. I was only on the medication for about three days and then hid all the rest of it in a handkerchief. About a week or so later, I disclosed that I still had all the medication. *Therefore I must be better, mustn't I? Because you thought I was on the medication and I wasn't* sort of thing. I never really took on board the fact that I had a mental illness and nobody pushed that on to me. Twelve years went by before I had another episode, after I'd come to New Zealand.

As I said, the first episode was triggered by a whole range of stressors. Similarly, in the second episode there were a whole lot of stressors. There was no further marijuana. Ever. But I'd had a third baby, I was in a new country, we were moving house, and I was trying to get to grips with the training in psychiatry which I'd just begun and which was enormously stressful.

I was very open. I wasn't stigmatised at that time, I didn't have the sense that *Oh God, I've got a mental illness, I'm somehow devalued* or, you know, *There's something wrong with me*. I thought, *Now this is rather amazing. I've had these psychotic episodes, I'm going to learn a lot from this*. I didn't feel frightened of the actual business of being psychotic, and I didn't have any sense of having a label on me. So I was very open with people, I talked about it with the consultants I worked for. I thought they would be genuinely interested.

When I was fully recovered I began to formulate an understanding of the possibility of recovery from psychotic illness. I thought what I've got is not schizophrenia but it's so similar to what people with schizophrenia suffer from. I could see if you could get the meaning of it and help someone to make sense of it, you could help them to recover. In a sense, looking back, I can see that I was beginning to grasp the possibility of early intervention.

I was very conscious of the need to make sense of the experience, and the need to help other people make sense of their experience. Not just talk to them in order to discover the phenomenology of their experience and put a diagnostic label on them, but to actually talk to them, to make a relationship with them, and understand them and their experience. That was what was missing from psychiatry when I was in training.

In subsequent years I had other episodes, very brief episodes, and I have gradually come to understand that I *do* have an illness and I *do* have a vulnerability. In some ways, it's become a lot more difficult for me because I'm no longer in denial about it.

I really didn't know that it could happen to me again. I felt well. *I don't have to let that happen again, it won't happen again.* And of course I've come across many patients who say and believe the same thing. I understand that now. Unfortunately it's not true, because it *can* happen again, and until you learn about your vulnerability and how to master it (which doesn't mean recovering from the vulnerability, it means living with it) you can't really recover. And that's what I *have* been able to do.

It's taken me a lot of learning experiences to come to that realisation, and it's not without sadness. In some ways I've probably become quite depressed recently in realising and having to take on board the reality of my continued vulnerability, and my need for continuous medication.

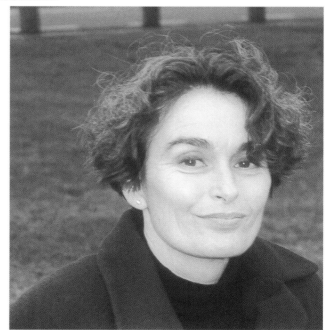

I've never seen myself as fitting into the DSM-IV diagnostic categories of mental illness.[1] I suppose you could say that I have multiple brief psychotic episodes. That would fit DSM-IV. I'm beginning to think there's a mood component, so maybe I have schizo-affective disorder. Maybe I have bipolar disorder, but it's hard, I don't fit perfectly into any category.

I don't think the categories *do* fit people. I think the categories are an attempt to understand a spectrum and make it into a categorical set. The diagnostic labels don't always help, and they can stigmatise. They don't even help with knowing what medications to use. It's becoming clear that people with schizophrenic illnesses often need mood stabilisers, and people with bipolar disorder sometimes need antipsychotics. I think it would be helpful to stop putting people in boxes. It's harder for people who've had this multiplicity of labels put on them to just take them off. We need better explanations.

I always believed that I had something to offer psy-

Photograph by Julie Leibrich

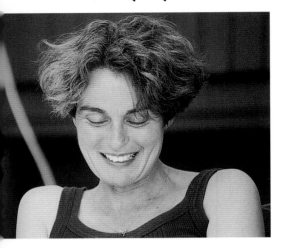

chiatry because of my personal understanding of psychosis. So you can imagine how shocked I was when in 1989 I was told out of the blue that I was not to be reappointed as a registrar. Effectively I was thrown out of the training scheme. Looking back, I think it was a discrimination against both my ideas and my illness. When I discussed my ideas about the possibility of recovery from psychosis with one of my senior colleagues, I was told that my understanding 'could be the most important breakthrough in psychiatry', and naïvely I believed it. Yet one of the reasons I was given for being thrown out was that my ideas were not acceptable. It was a paradox. It didn't make any sense.

But I suspect that concern about my illness was also implicated. At the time, I didn't realise I was being discriminated against. It's only in retrospect that I've recognised that.

I feel that what happened to me in psychiatry impacted on me hugely. It made my illness much worse. My illness would not have got so bad had it not happened to me. At the point I realised I was being excluded from psychiatry I was devastated, I was totally devastated. *Apart from my children and my husband, how can I go on living? What is the meaning of my life? I thought my life was about making a contribution to psychiatry, now I can't even darken their doors.*

One day, I gave some thought to killing myself. It wasn't over any prolonged time, but it was just one day I thought, I imagined …. I talked to my husband about how desperate I was feeling, and he made an interesting suggestion – that I go and talk to a pastor.

In the last nine years I have come to recognise God and Jesus as a reality. It's become a very important aspect of my reality that has helped in my recovery and survival. I've no doubt about that at all. I know that has been a major part of restoring my sense of my self. It's made it possible for me to see my own broken-ness, but also know my own value and worth. I'm sure people can do that without a Christian perspective, it was just where my path lead me.

A Scripture that has really spoken to me is that *God's grace is sufficient for me, and His strength was made perfect in my weakness.* So it's okay for me to be weak, because in my weakness He's made strong, and I can do God's work out of my own broken-ness. So it's really cut across my own grandiosity. I no longer have to feel like I'm going to make the most important breakthrough in psychiatry.

The other image that I'd had during one of my psychotic episodes was that someone was the Devil. I'd had images of evil and satanic influence. It didn't make sense in my world view, but for some reason it seemed like that was reality when I was psychotic. So it was very helpful to discover that Satan does exist in the Christian world view, as an understanding of where evil comes from. That we're not fighting human enemies, we're fighting a war in the spirit. So I saw that what had happened to me in psychiatry was the result of a spiritual battle, not a personal battle.

Now, I'm part of a church. I have a lot of personal support. I have a prayer partner and friends who share my world view. I go to my church regularly, and I pray and read Scriptures every day. It gives me strength.

After coming into Christianity, I felt called again to go back into psychiatry, to complete my training, or to do this piece of work that I had in my heart to do – which was to demonstrate that loving relationship is at the root of recovery.

I seemed to have a special aptitude working with people with really serious treatment-resistant psychotic illness, where other people couldn't begin to make a relationship. I'd had enough experience clinically to know that if I stayed in a relationship with people, and helped them to make sense of their experience, they began to recover. I felt called to complete my training so that I could do this piece of work.

This was in 1994, and things had changed by then because there was an awareness of discrimination and stigma. As soon as I reapplied to go back into psychiatry I was accepted, no questions asked. Nobody asked about my illness, or about what had happened in the past about my ideas. There was no discussion about it whatsoever. It was as if nothing had happened, and that was just as traumatising to me as when I had been thrown out. Once again, it didn't make any sense. I was paradoxed and paradoxed again.

Being so vulnerable and so sensitive, immediately after they'd accepted me back I became psychotic again. Anyway I recovered and they still accepted me back, knowing my vulnerability. I've always been very pleased about that, because it means that it's all out in the open now and there's no discrimination against me, thank goodness.

The only discrimination I've felt since then is my own self-stigmatisation. You know, a real questioning of my own worth and value as someone with a mental illness. That's been really devastating for me. It's to do with the validation of the person, in the sense of who you are in relation to someone else. That you have worth and value to somebody else. I think part of what happens with psychotic illness is you lose your connection. Well, not just with psychotic illness *per se*, but with the stigmatisation that comes along with psychosis.

I didn't experience this at the beginning. In fact I experienced a height-

[7]To keep me from becoming conceited because of these surpassingly great revelations, there was given me a thorn in my flesh, a messenger of Satan, to torment me. [8]Three times I pleaded with the Lord to take it away from me. [9]But he said to me, 'My grace is sufficient for you, for my power is made perfect in weakness.' Therefore I will boast all the more gladly about my weaknesses, so that Christ's power may rest on me. [10]That is why, for Christ's sake, I delight in weaknesses, in insults, in hardships, in persecutions, in difficulties. For when I am weak, then I am strong.

Corinthians 12, verses 7–10

The opening of my essay which won first prize in **Australasian Psychiatry's** Essay Competition in 1995, and appeared in the December 1995 issue of the journal. In the editorial it was noted that 'four of the five judges chose Dr Randall's entry as the winner and the fifth had it in second place.' Also that all three prize-winning entries came from New Zealand authors, going on to say 'The future of New Zealand psychiatry appears to be in good hands'.

ened sense of connectedness with people and with life and with the meaning of life initially, so it's obviously not *just* about psychosis.

But when you're stigmatised I think you feel like you don't belong any more, and you don't matter any more, and that you're not to be taken seriously. I have really questioned, *Am I credible, am I worth listening to?* and I think you need to recover that in a relationship, you need someone to enable you to experience again that you have validity and value. You're not an invalid. You're not invalid.

You have worth, value, validity, credibility. You *mean* something to someone else. I don't think you can discover that except in a relationship. Two friends, who are psychiatrists, really helped me with that. I felt my calling was in psychiatry and they really helped to validate me again. Saying that my ideas do make sense.

The other thing that really helped was that I won an essay competition in 1995 – actually won it on my birthday. That was an extraordinary affirmation because in the editorial of the journal in which it was published it said clearly the future of New Zealand psychiatry is in good hands.[2] It was such an affirmation, and that was an important part of my recovery, because it gave me back my sense of my own value and credibility.

Another thing that has been really important to me is that I have a very

'Although science is an essential part of psychiatry, it is not its essence.'

Dr John Ellard, AM

John Ellard's challenging statement stimulates a sequence of questions for discussion. To begin, what is science, what is its relationship with psychiatry, and what is the difference between an essence and an essential part? Perhaps finding answers to these questions might go some way to defining all that psychiatry is. The Concise Oxford Dictionary definitions are as follows:

Science n. A branch of knowledge conducted on objective principles involving the systematised observation of, and experiment with, phenomena; systematic and formulated knowledge.

Essence n. The indispensable quality or element; identifying a thing or determining a thing, or determining its character; fundamental nature or inherent characteristics; and extract obtained by distillation etc; perfume, scent; and abstract entity; the reality underlying a phenomenon.

Essential a. Absolutely necessary; indispensable; fundamentally basic; of or constituting, the essence of a person or thing.

Does Dr Ellard imply that there is a single most fundamental essence of psychiatry, which is not science, and if so, what is it? Or perhaps the implication is that there are many essential parts of psychiatry, of which science is only one? Why make this statement? Does it imply that there are some psychiatrists who might mistakenly believe that science is indeed the essence of psychiatry, or the essence of anything?

In this essay, these questions are addressed, and an attempt made to substantiate the notion that psychiatry does indeed have a fundamental essence. Although it cannot as yet be stated as fact, my hypothesis is that this essence lies in the relationship between psychiatrist and patient. …

close friendship with a woman who is a doctor and has a diagnosis of bipolar disorder, so there are a number of things we have in common. I know I've been of major value to her, and she's been of major value to me. Finding another person who I can touch base with has been really really important. I don't want to minimise that.

My husband and children have been just brilliant. That's been very restoring. I thank my faith as much as anything for the restoration of that. Having that close relationship and that trust and that support. I know it hasn't been easy for them.

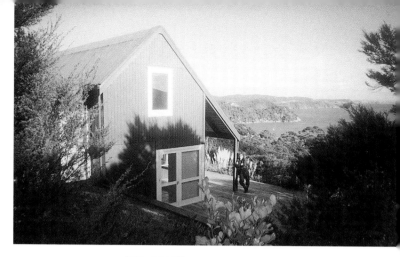

The holiday house.

I think what helps me is just being very conscious of what's happening to me, being able to reflect on it, being able to reality-test with a whole gallery of people so that I've got lots of points of reference to anchor me.

I take medication, which is equally important, and I've come to realise that I can't get my cognition (thinking) straight if my affect (feelings) isn't straight. And I can't get my affect straight except by using medication when I'm stressed. I've come to realise that at times I need medication in order to feel calm and peaceful.

I have my own personal psychiatrist who I go and see regularly. I've kept in touch with her through all these years, and I always let her know if I'm taking medication or stopping medication or whatever. She hasn't really helped me understand my illness or come to terms with it or recover, but I've really appreciated her. Just because I know she's there. And it's been particularly useful for my husband to know she was there.

Then there are other things that I do. I walk my dog with my husband. And I make sure I have lots of rest – I'm learning to cut down on the amount of demands I make on myself. I've had to learn to know my limits. And we bought a holiday house recently, which is going to be a wonderful place of retreat and restoration.

Postscript

It wasn't easy to decide to tell my story in this book but I want to be part of the process that leads to reducing discrimination and stigma against people with mental illness. If this book can do that, then I'm happy.

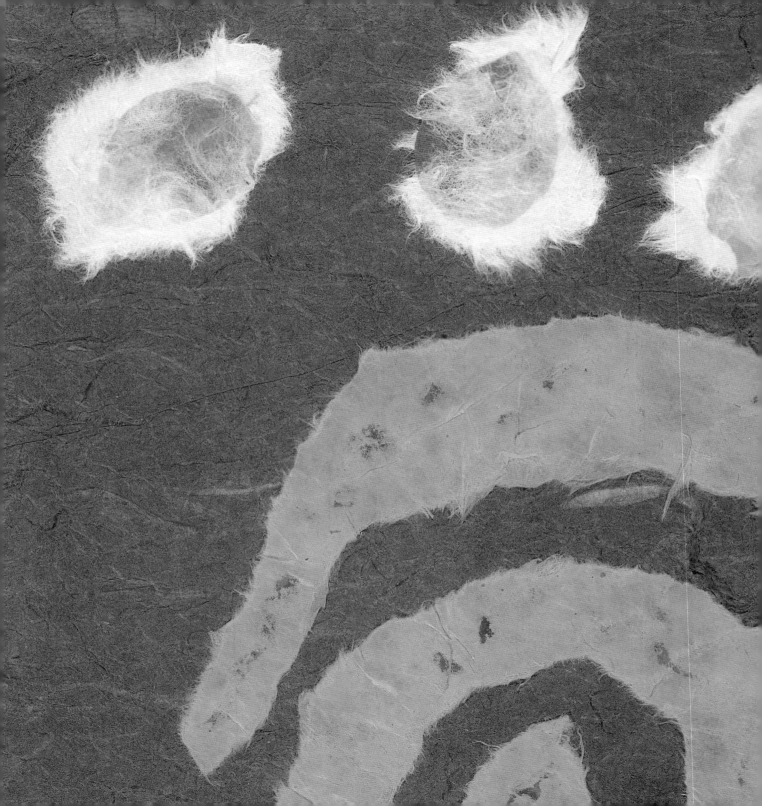

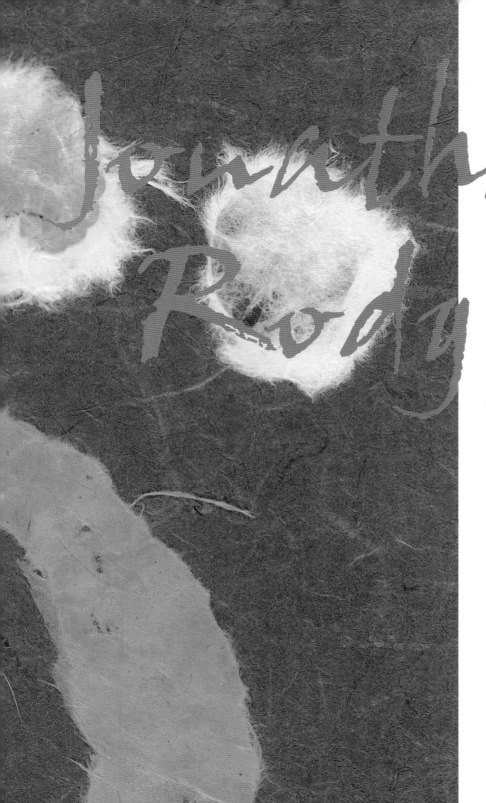

It's like a journey into
the light, says

Jonathan Rodgers

Jonathan is thirty-eight, and studying for his BA in Visual Art and Design at EIT in the Hawke's Bay. He and his partner, Kay, have a young son called Zachary (also known as Dynamite!).

You can be feeling fine and then all of a sudden it's a shadow. You sort of walk out of the sun into the shadow. You don't know you're doing it and suddenly you feel the coolness of this shadow. And with depression it permeates you, gets right through to you.

I've suffered for years with depression, but only recently, in the last year or so, I've acknowledged it and sought professional help through my GP. I was at an absolute low ebb. I didn't think I was ever going to come into the sunshine again. Because that's what's it's like for me when I feel depressed, I just go into this immense darkness and you're getting swallowed up by a big hole. There's nothing to grip on to and nothing to climb out with and it gets pretty desperate.

If the depression came on really bad, I wouldn't maintain appointments. I just let everything slide. Then I'd just come back out of it, and I'd be okay and just carry on as if nothing had happened. I'd never mention missed appointments and things like that, and people never seemed to raise it with me. But, you know, when you do that time and time again, people tend to stop inviting you to do things. So it has taken a toll, in a way.

There are times when you feel like you just don't want to go on any more and you think about ways of killing yourself. *What is the easiest way? What's not going to hurt me?* I have contemplated doing stupid things to myself, but I think that that is as far as I would ever take it, just thinking about it, just the desperation of it at the moment.

I knew how to manage it myself, really. When I got depressed, I was totally isolated. I would shut myself away, not see people, not visit or answer the door. As the years went on I realised that it was a process, and if I could wait it out, it would fade and I would start feeling okay again, functioning, feeling social, and wanting to see people.

I was always afraid to label myself. I didn't want a label. If anything, I wanted to be labelled as brilliant and creative. I didn't want to be labelled as depressed and down. So all those years of going through that.

I suppose my all-time worst low was when my grandparents died. They were my last connection with family. That was total severance of love and acceptance. There was quite an alienation from my mother with her remarrying when I was ten years old, and that alienation has grown over the years. It hasn't healed or changed, it has continued to get worse. I was never able to talk to my mother about my depression, because she refused to recognise it.

When I left school, I went to live with my grandparents. I'd spent five years with my mother and stepfather, and I'd say it would be the most torturous time in my life – the least understood, the least accepted, the least trusted, the least all these things. Then I went to my grandparents and it was great. It was all the love and support and stuff that any young person could want. And life seemed to be really normal. And I did lots of different jobs – in a supermarket, a construction gang, then at the railways.

At that stage (I was about seventeen) I really knew 'my artist within' was screaming out. I was drawing and I was painting. I think that's when I knew I had depression – when I first started seriously believing that I was an artist.

When I was twenty-three, I was an angry young man and I was working as a shearer. Working all over New Zealand. You know, working hard and playing hard and drinking lots of alcohol and things like that. I loved that lifestyle, loved the job, it never gave me any time to think about depression.

But my self-destructive urges were

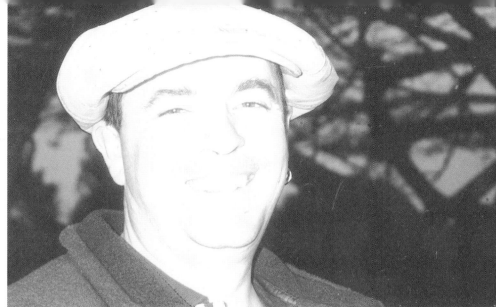

Photograph by Julie Leibrich

doing mad things, you know – spur of the moment things, really dangerous things. Driving and riding motorcycles really fast and doing ridiculous things on them. And standing on a cliff-top with a blanket holding myself against a gale-force wind. Just because it was there, and I could feel the strength of the wind, and I knew it wasn't going to let me go. I never once thought that I would fall off, and the feeling of exhilaration while I was doing it was immense. It was overwhelming.

I first came to Wellington when I was twenty-nine and I started work at Vincents.[1] I wanted to work with people and help people who couldn't help themselves. I worked there for three years as assistant co-ordinator, and my main job was running and organising workshops and tutoring, and helping people with creative problems. So it was really a problem-solving job. I inspired people, I hope – and I was inspired by the place as well.

Vincents was for me, workwise, my high point. I felt like I was giving something really good back. Also helping and understanding. Vincents is just there with open arms for everybody. That's what I loved about it when I worked there. It wasn't just a drop-in centre for 'the psychiatrically disabled', it was a drop-in centre for the whole community of unemployed people in the city. And that breaks down a lot of barriers, because people who are just unemployed and have no mental illness, or history or inkling of it, get to see what it's like for people who suffer with depression and schizophrenia every day.

That was when I first started with the dog motif as an artist. Because I felt all these people at Vincents were all terribly marginalised. They were dogs, treated like dogs, kicked like dogs, you know, occasional pat-on-the-head sort of thing. That's really where the dog theme came from. People marginalised. Mongrels of society.

I think society is afraid of mental illness. Probably for a lot of the reasons I never wanted to admit my *own* depression. Society thinks people with mental illness have no will, have nothing to offer any more, have lost their effectiveness in society.

People at Vincents showed me that they are working at the level that they *can* work at. Everybody in society is aiming for their peak, and no one wants less than their peak. We are in this thing together and some of us are depressed. Some of us are sportspeople and some of us are artists, some of us are poets, some of us are musicians, some of us are politicians. But it's when we start saying because I'm a politician I'm better than you, or because I'm an artist I'm better than you … If you have this 'better than you' mentality it isolates you from the rest of the world, the rest of life. You become so blinkered.

But life is full of strange and wonderful things, and in a sense depression is a gift for people. When I was at Vincents, I could never admit to myself that I was depressed. I fitted in there really well. And I know why *now* – because I was just like them, I *am* just like them. I get depression.

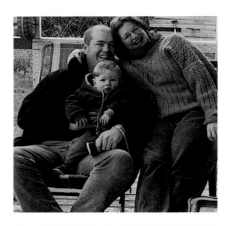

Me, Zachary and Kay.

Over the years I've done therapies and stuff, but I didn't really understand I had depression. I did a co-counselling course and it was wonderful for me. It took me out of my angry young man phase. I started being more philosophical and practical about the way I sometimes felt, not letting it grind me into dust but hopefully polishing me a little bit more. Every time that I survived it, I felt a little bit more polished, a little bit more able to cope with it next time.

That course was just amazing. It opened myself up to my feelings and examining them – saying, you know, *this is how I feel and this is what I think*. I started becoming less angry and more productive with my anger, driving that into my work. I was determined to become an artist and to exhibit regularly, and that's really been my driving force for the last twenty years. It's like a journey into the light.

When Zachary was born, I just thought that was the greatest thing in the world that ever happened to me. It was amazing. He was so beautiful and perfect and Kay was a great mother and it was another level in our relationship. But I was having a really hard time going through all that, having down feelings about what my role was as a parent, being in and out of work and an unreliable provider, and all that sort of stuff. So the depression seemed to get a lot worse and I wasn't dealing with it.

I was getting more angry and resentful because I didn't feel anyone understood what was going on for me. I did talk to friends about it, but they always said, *You're all right*, you know, slap on the back, and I'd just sort of take that and carry on.

It was a big step for me to get professional help, because it was something I had hidden. I didn't feel particularly good about being depressed. I wanted to be just 'normal', I suppose. That's why I tried to hide it all the time.

Zachary was my reason for looking for professional help, because I had a lot more at stake. It wasn't just me any more. I had Kay and Zachary. So I saw my GP and went on Prozac for a while and that helped, I suppose. I felt good that I was getting recognition for what I was feeling and it helped me get out of the real downer that I was in. But as soon as I started feeling better again, I didn't want to take the medication any more because I was having lots of really vivid dreams and disturbed sleep, so I'd wake up feeling tired in the morning as well.

I went and talked to the people at Community Mental Health but I didn't think I got the help I really needed, because their first answer was medication, and I've always been resistant to that. I also met a psychiatrist through them, but it was a non-event, really. I thought he was there just filling in his day. I didn't feel he had any compassion or understanding. I thought I would be able to understand what my thinking was all about and try to replace the circuits and cross over the switches and play around with it in that sense, and try and stop it. I didn't feel any resolution. When I talked to him he just seemed to say, *Well, of course you are depressed, this is the sort of life you had, blah, blah, blah*. Me suffering the depression, I can't write it off like that and just say it was because of this or because of that.

That's when I realised that they couldn't help me. Only I could help me, of course, because all depression is unique to the individual and I can't expect that other people can find resolution for me. That's where

One half of my smile.

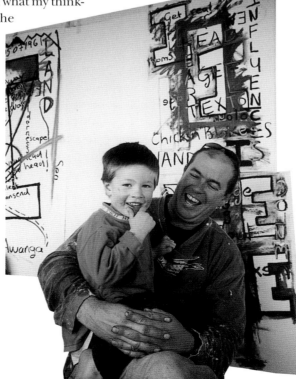

I get my strength from – from knowing that I can create my own solutions and that I'm not incapable. I suppose I know now that it just can't be stopped, it's just not a stoppable thing. It's just there and it's like a little gremlin sitting on my shoulder.

I think about depression a lot. I think about not wanting to get depressed again and always thinking it's just around the corner. But it seems to have changed. It's no longer months of totally down. It's almost like I can have a bad day and a day is okay. I can handle a bad *day*. I'm so relieved when I get up and I am not feeling depressed. And if I feel better today it's great; if I don't, I just ride with it.

I get a lot of self-esteem from the work I do. I get immense joy from the act of creating, making, discovering, and that's exciting, but when the depression arrives you can still be doing those things but none of the excitement is there. None of the enjoyment, the pleasure, the passion. Your passion gets sucked out of you. The passion seems to be taken over by the depression. It's almost like depression is the total opposite of passion.

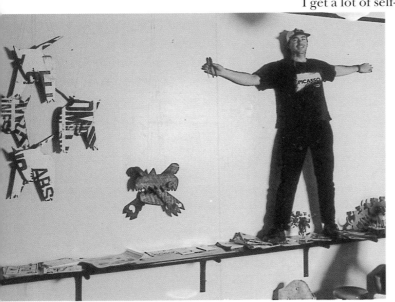

Dog images.

I had a good friend, Mark Whyte, and I had my very first exhibition with Mark. We travelled around New Zealand and toured in public bars. We just showed our work in all these public bars and we had a ball doing it – it was great. Mark was always a really good sounding board for me, and I used to talk to him about when I felt depressed – about not creating and stuff – and he'd say things like, W*ell, you've just got to allow your creativity to go in its own cycle, it's a natural process* and things like that. So I started looking at my depression in a seasonal sense.

I actually found my year would be broken up just like the seasons, summer, winter, autumn and spring. The spring was when the flush was on and there was lots of energy happening and lots of ideas percolating, and then the summer would come on and be just the most wonderfully creative time. Then the autumn would be the start of the depression and the energy dropping off, and then the winter would be the total despair of the depression. It would be a yearly cycle and I expected to be like this or that for so many months and it just seemed to work that way and I don't know why.

I've always had strong feelings and been sensitive to situations and things that are happening around me. Very aware, hyper-aware almost, of things around me. And it's quite a wonderful thing. I can be talking to people and say, *Oh did you see that?* and they don't see stuff. Or I'm talking about things that people don't even think about. That's why I said it's a gift because you get opportunities to see a little bit more of life, in a more raw state or whatever.

It's just the darkness I don't like. I was doing a bit of writing a while ago about what was inside me when I was depressed, and it was this little wee boy in this dark dark room with no windows, no doors. It's like total rejection. It's like, imagining you're a baby and you're screaming and you're crying for your mother and she is just never coming. You're just in this darkness. That's what I fear about depression. That's what I fear. Because when I get *that* depressed, there is no contact with the outside world. There is no warmth. No joy. That's what I fear about it, the removal of all those beautiful things, the ability to experience beauty.

It seems to me that it goes hand-in-hand almost with being a creative person. Being creative, the creativity, that's how I love myself. That's how I say to myself *I'm okay.* That's where I get meaning from. Being creative, you're actually allowed to be on your own and be quiet and have this reflection. So in a sense, for me, it is not such a hard thing because I do see that seasonal aspect of my creativity and my cycle of life.

I've decided to go to Napier next year to the art school. It's a BA degree. I've just got a lot of stuff in me that I'm not articulating, that I really need to do. If I don't go and do it now, and I don't get the tools to articulate myself in the way that I want, I don't think I'll ever fully mature as an artist. I think having the structure of the degree will really help me a lot. I suppose, in a way, it might be a combative tool against the blackness of the depression. I might be able to get in and actually draw something out of that blackness.

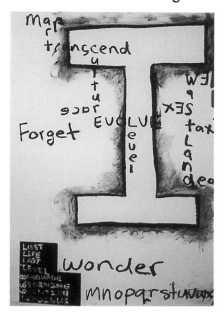

I wonder

Postscript

This year, in February I started art school with much trepidation and anticipation. In the short four months I have been there, the anticipation has been more than fulfilled and the strength that I am gathering at art school is more than I could have hoped for. The trepidation has faded into insignificance and turned to relish for the challenge. I look forward to completing my degree – with honours!

I no longer am who I think I am,
I am not the plaything of my
thoughts

Nietzche

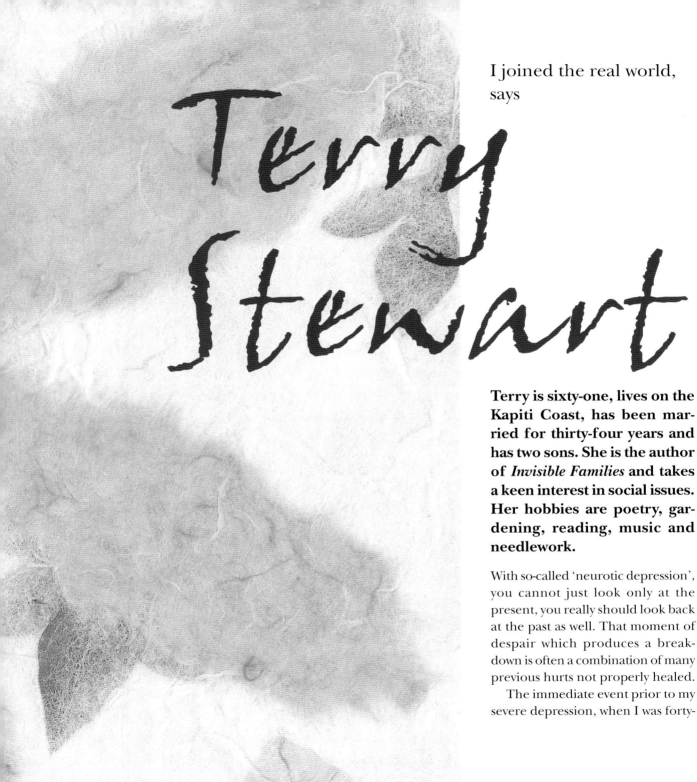

I joined the real world,
says

Terry Stewart

Terry is sixty-one, lives on the Kapiti Coast, has been married for thirty-four years and has two sons. She is the author of *Invisible Families* and takes a keen interest in social issues. Her hobbies are poetry, gardening, reading, music and needlework.

With so-called 'neurotic depression', you cannot just look only at the present, you really should look back at the past as well. That moment of despair which produces a breakdown is often a combination of many previous hurts not properly healed.

The immediate event prior to my severe depression, when I was forty-

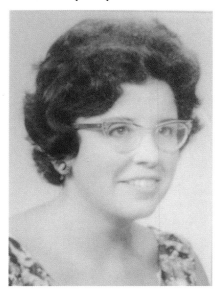

As a young woman.

four, was a hysterectomy. It didn't go smoothly and I had internal bleeding and a great deal of pain and other problems. Then my wound went septic and I had more bleeding and went back for more surgery. I was in a high state of anxiety.

In retrospect, I had had anxiety attacks for some months before surgery, but hadn't recognised this. The hysterectomy was the last straw. Looking further back, I can see I was depressed from childhood, for several reasons. I feel this was partly inherited.

In particular, I had been teased and nagged about being overweight, which was again partly genetic. I was never bulimic or anything like that, but I ate for comfort. And then when I was twelve, I caught polio and I couldn't exercise much, which meant more weight again.

In those days nothing was done for anything but the physical trauma of polio. In the hospital I was friends with a girl in an iron-lung, and one morning she wasn't there. We knew she had died but nobody said anything. We waited for our turn to die, and it didn't happen. We were told we were lucky and to get on with life, which of course was essentially right. But we lived with the fear and guilt. You see, nothing was explained.

Many of us became achieving perfectionists.[1] So I coped by being 'better then abled' when in fact I had moderately severe disabilities which I deliberately hid.

I suffered most as a teenager in not being able to wear the latest shoes and so on – winkle-pickers, for example. Everything I wore was clunky and hopelessly out of date. I used to cry in every shoe shop in Queen Street. I wore glasses and was shy. Boys would smile, then see my hand and limp, and look away.

I was twenty-seven before I married and found someone who could see past all that. Then I was whisked from the city to a farm, a huge challenge. When we discussed having children, the doctor said, *You're too overweight* (I was thirteen stone) and he put me on amphetamines (speed!) to diet.

After both my babies, I had depression. The first time, it wasn't diagnosed. I just battled on. The second time my GP gave me valium.

In the nine years from 1966, when my first son was born prematurely, I had four minor operations, a severe infective illness, and a second baby.

I can see that all this was a cry for help. I just wasn't coping. So I was taking time out. In a way, I was looking after myself. That's what I think it was.

At the time of the hysterectomy and also because of the polio, I had severe backache. I received no support for that whatsoever. When I had to go back into hospital for the second time, I remember not sleeping, and sitting in the middle of the night and dry-retching, and nobody taking the least bit of notice.

One morning, about five days later, the staff nurse came round and stood at the end of the bed and said, *Well, what's all this about, then?* I was confused and said the first thing that came into my head, *My uncle's just died in Britain.* And she said, *Oh, is that all,* and walked away.

It was all a chapter of accidents: fear of authority, sleep deprivation, lack of knowledge, and poor care. If only someone had stepped in then and said, *This woman is unduly anxious and sliding into post-operative depression,* it might all have been stopped and I would not have lost the equivalent of six years of my life.

When I went home, I didn't get any better. The agitation grew and became free-floating. I couldn't sleep, I couldn't read, I couldn't sit still for long, I couldn't listen to music, I couldn't talk to people. People would visit, but three minutes of chat was enough. I'd disappear and lie on the bed again.

In the mornings, I'd dry-retch before managing to shower. Then I'd lie down again and cry or stare into space. By about the middle of the afternoon I'd think, *The children are coming home from school, I must get up and make some dinner.* I'd go to the freezer, look at the meat and couldn't decide what to do with it, then cry some more.

It must have been terrible for Ron. He hung in there every step of the way. It nearly pushed him to the edge. He was so good. I've heard of people with severe depression whose families have just walked away. They couldn't cope. He is one of the most loyal, dearest, kindest of men.

It was a slow descent into hell. There's no other way to put it. After nearly four months, I threatened to hang myself. Then I was sent to a private hospital and given antidepressants and tranquillisers, which I needed. These knocked me flat and then brought me round again. After three weeks I went home.

Then a worse hell took over. I thought I had been in hell, but then I went deeper. That's the reality of it. Over the next four years, I became dependent on ativan. Now I know that ativan is a benzodiazapine tranquilliser, which shouldn't be used long term for people with damage to the central nervous system, like me.

I lost all sense of who I was. I lost my spirituality, I lost my creativity, I lost my sexuality, and I became a nothing. I became a shell of a person, and it was the most annihilating experience. It was like being part of the walking dead.

By late 1983, I'd asked to come off ativan but my specialist said, *No, no,*

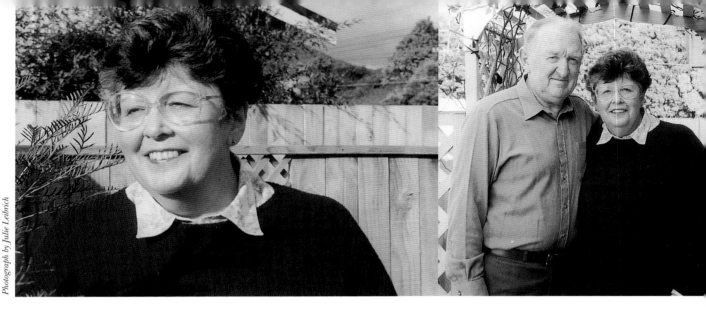

Right: Ron and I.

you need them. My GP held my hand and said, *Terry, I wouldn't hurt you, I am doing the best I can for you.* And although I questioned them several times, they just gave me more.

My parents, like Ron, were also loving and supportive, but in 1986, my dear mum died suddenly. She was buried on my birthday, which nobody had thought about. I missed her dreadfully but was too drugged to grieve properly.

By January of 1987, I was twelve tablets a day: four anafranil for depression, six 2.5 mg of ativan for anxiety, and two 2.5 mg of halcion for sleeping. And I became progressively less able to function.

Then I had a terrifying episode of hallucinatory depersonalisation. I was feeling dreadful one hot afternoon and I went to take a shower. But I just sat down fully dressed in its cool space. And at some point began banging my head on the side of the shower box. Later, when I looked up above the shower rail, I saw myself floating against the ceiling looking down. I felt utterly paralysed. It must have been over an hour before Ron found me and got me to move.

After that, I insisted on other advice and saw the psychologist at the local public hospital. I asked him, *Am I going mad?* because I was afraid I'd end up in Carrington.[2] He was actually the first person who really listened to me. He said, *I think you have ativan dependency* and sent me to a psychiatrist who agreed. And they took me off it.

This began eighteen months of an even deeper hell. The withdrawal symptoms took me back to being suicidal, and at one point the psychiatrist wanted to hospitalise me. I couldn't face the psych ward, yet couldn't bear to be alone. With the support of friends I pulled through at home. They rostered themselves for the week so I wasn't by myself while Ron was at work.

At their worst, the withdrawal symptoms came in waves of intense anxiety, panic and dread, depression, palpitations, and severe headaches, with a tension band which didn't lift for a single day for over four months. Vivid horror nightmares, excessive sweating, flu-like aches and pains, nausea and sinus problems.

That all took a full year to get over, and even then, I was getting flashbacks at night, like nightmares, but they gradually got less and less until they disappeared. So I never underestimate somebody who fights off tranquilliser dependency or drug addictions. All the family suffered greatly and we lost a lot financially.

I reckon I cried every single day for a year. Every time anyone came near me I bawled. All the anguish and grief from the past that I'd never let go of just came out by the bucketful. I didn't think I'd ever stop crying. The boys, of course, found it extremely difficult. I mean, their mother was falling apart. Mother, who'd been so strong. They tried hard to understand and help.

My friends were marvellous. One friend I remember came round when I was sitting on the bed, just crying really. And she lovingly said, *It'll come right, you will bloom gently again where you are.* She was so nice, walking around me, dusting the furniture, saying, *Don't worry about it, just let it happen.* Others brought soup and stuff for the children to eat. I remember that was really wonderful, very supportive. Only a couple of friends faded away.

They didn't judge. They didn't say, *Pull your socks up,* which is the worst sort of thing to say to someone. When you're in the depths, you can't, you can only live through it. Later on I was able to see little areas of hope and gradually it built up.

Books have helped. I have read an enormous amount and found one or two books along the way which have helped a lot.[3] I think that even if you read a book and you don't really understand it, there will be little gems in it which will hit you.

By 1988, I was able to work part-time with what's now called the Northland Mental Health Trust. Looking back, I can see that it was part of my recovery to work with people whose problems were worse than my own. I learnt so much from their sheer guts and strength.

I helped run a support group for people with manic depression, and I edited a newsletter and wrote information pamphlets. It was so valuable

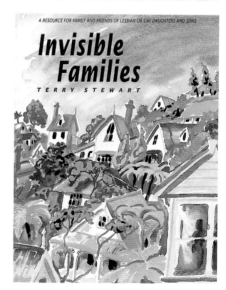

Invisible Families. Originally published by New Women's Press, 1993.

A RESOURCE FOR FAMILY AND FRIENDS OF LESBIAN OR GAY DAUGHTERS AND SONS

Invisible Families

TERRY STEWART

Modern Poetry is difficult

I was raised
with verses of Pooh Bear,
The same of Little Brain
who floated, blackly as a cloud
and hummed aloud
to scare the bees.

I loved early
'Earth has not anything
to show more fair',
 Old ships sailing 'like swans asleep',
Daffodils in 'sprightly dance',
Which was not chance.

For I was taught
that metre matters;
That lines should scan
and alliteration
underscores the scheme
of lofty narrative theme.

Modern poetry
omits
develops scantily
does not punctuate
has odd adjectives in places odd
leaves gaps
that do not stimulate
the imagination.
Starkness is its soul
Brevity its watchword.

My heart yearns
for the Victorians
and Rupert Brooke.

Terry Georgina Stewart

because it took out the self-pity which had started to creep in. While there, I did a two-year course, called Caring Education,[4] from the ASTU at Massey. That was great. It was a formal exam and I got a B+. I was really very pleased with myself and felt that I had achieved something. That gave me confidence and I decided to do a year's course in journalism.

Around this time, there were a lot of extra stresses in my life. We took on the care of Ron's parents – both disabled and in their nineties. Also, our son came out to us as being gay, which wasn't easy to deal with. It meant a rethink of much misinformation we had picked up. In fact, it led to me writing my book *Invisible Families*.[5]

One day I had heard Wendy Harrex from New Women's Press talk about publishing, and Wendy had some of her books there, including things on overweight and non-fiction things, and I said to her, *You know, you should get someone to write a book for parents of gay and lesbian children.* She never missed a beat, she just looked me in the eye and said, *Why don't you write it yourself?*

The contract for writing this book came just as I had started the journalism course, which meant that while studying I was researching for the book, and being swept into active campaigning for the Human Rights law amendments.[6]

Because of all the stress I went back on a mild antidepressant for the next three years. The book was launched in 1993, Ron's parents went into other care, we moved to the Kapiti coast and renovated a house.

But by late 1996, I still wasn't coping well. I've learnt the signs and learnt not to ignore them. When tunes I've heard keep going over and over in my head or if I keep waking up at 4am, I know I've got to slow up. I've got to cut back on what I'm doing and calm down. To not force things and be kind to myself.

When I get the feeling that I'm ploughing through cotton wool and might drop off an edge, or if I start cutting myself off from other people, I know it's time to do something about it.

My GP suggested a different antidepressant – Prozac. It was wonderful. I felt the best since I was thirteen. After a year I slowly came off it. A year later I started slipping again and I'm now back on Prozac. I'm feeling really strong and I'm happy to stay on it.

I think my taking it is no different from a diabetic taking insulin to be well. Having been across that chemical edge within my brain, I feel that edge is there. It's like being an alcoholic. I don't think I can ever say that I am fully recovered in the sense that I still have a predisposition to depressive illness, which for me, I feel, has a hormonal component. One day, there may be a cure. To be involved and busy is to live. So there has to be some compromise, which for me, is medication.

I think that when I was first depressed, I was afraid to tell people. I was ashamed of what I thought was a further flaw, and I felt vulnerable. I was so nicely middle-class, Anglican, very sheltered, never questioning authorities. I dated late, I did my overseas experience late, married late, and had children late. I've never really been in step with my peers, didn't get the chance to further my education and was often very lonely.

I've learnt heaps and done so much that I never dreamt of, through having a breakdown and joining the real world. I've met terrific, real people – those who, by hard experience, know life is not fair or perfect. To understand that no matter how good I am, life is not always going to be good in return – this was a true gift. I've left behind the imposed guilt and fear of not quite measuring up for home, church, or school. Any God knows I've done my best from my genetic basis, with the talent such as I've been given, or what I knew at the time.

I'm more aware of what I am, what I have, and of the precious things life offers. As Melody Beatty says in *Journey to the Heart*:[7]

> Believing in life means it's okay to let go. We can trust where we've been. We trust where we're going. And we're right where we need to be now. Believe in Life.

I don't recommend a breakdown to anyone. But for me, the outcomes of my breakdown have been so positive.

Opposite: A poem of mine, 'Modern Poetry is Difficult', published in *Spirit of Kapiti: Kapiti Poems 8.* (Kapiti Creative Publishing Group Inc. in association with Steele Roberts, 1999.)

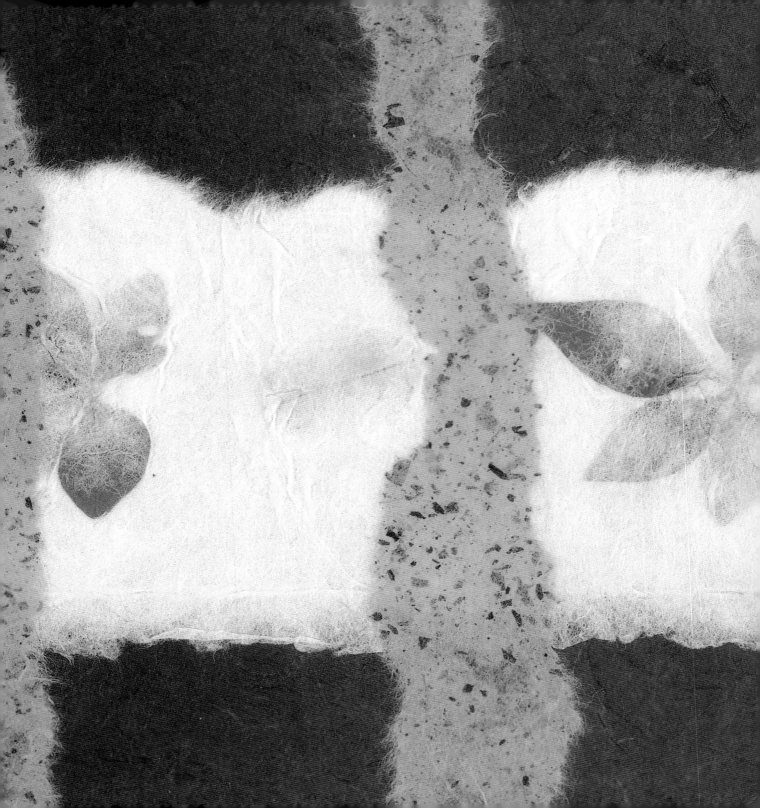

You have to protect your affect, says

Alasdair Russell

Alasdair was an engineer until manic depression changed the course of his life. He was devoted to improving the lives of people with manic depression and at the time of his death was setting up the West Auckland Manic Depression Information Trust.

I can remember being picked up once on the way to Tauranga. I was hitchhiking. This chap (I'm sure he didn't realise that sitting in his car was a nutter) said, *You know, these people who come out of these institutions, they should never let them out. Lock them up, that's what I say.* I didn't dare say that I was one of them.

A lot of people don't understand the word manic, or mania. You get an incredible sense of power and energy. The way people identify a manic state is, first of all, you have pressure of speech. And if you know that that's happening to you, you can slow your voice down, you can modulate it a bit more, you can pace yourself out. People wouldn't know that you've got a racing mind, you're conversing with them normally. If they are perceiving only a normal conversation, they've got no clues, no insight into the fact that inside that brain of yours, there's a fire going on.

It began for me when I was about nineteen. I made a trip to America and I didn't know what had happened. I went by myself to a strange country. From the time I started the flight, something had happened to me. It was an excited state. By the time I got to America I was basically out of my tree, but I didn't know what it was. No one had said to me, *Look, this is obviously what you are suffering from.* I thought it was something that no one had ever talked about, you know. I had never had that experience before. I was manic. I did some bizarre things. I thought some bizarre things. I cut the trip short by a week, flew back to New Zealand, and thought everyone knew what had been going on in the States. But of course nobody did.

After that, I was having mood swings but mainly depressive mood swings. I wasn't suffering from the mania so much but I was having these bouts of depression. The doctor at Air New Zealand, where I worked, said to me, *Look, you'll have to go and see a psychiatrist,* and I thought, *This is crazy, I don't need any of this attention, I'm not mad, what are you doing this to me for?* They sent me to see someone but I never told him about this manic experience. I didn't know what mania was, I didn't know about manic depression, I never told him I had this elated experience.

I got married in December 1975 but my illness put a great stress on my relationship with my wife. Some days I would get so depressed that I couldn't get out of bed. And a few months later I was manic and went and bought a $10,000 vehicle that I couldn't afford. So I was admitted to Carrington. I was kept there for a few weeks and told I had manic depression. Lithium was the drug prescribed.

I went up to see Air New Zealand again, because I still had a fixation about that company. Then I went to the basement and pinched their mail van, and started driving it around town. I was off my face, I was off my trolley. The police picked me up and I got thrown in the Wharf Police Station that evening about five o'clock.

While they were interviewing me and going through my bag, I tore out a hole in the ceiling of the cell, broke out all the plaster, put my jacket

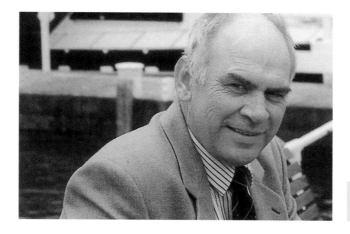

At the Best Practice
Conference, Tauranga, 1997.

down on the floor so they couldn't hear the noise of the plaster coming down, and climbed up into the attic, into a granary chute. The police came into the room and they didn't look up. They just looked down and they saw all this crap on the floor, and said, *Christ, he's gone!* And I said, *No, it's all right, I'm up here.* I called out from about twenty feet above them, you see.

I ended up going before the Court. I spent a night in Mount Eden, and they suspected there was something seriously wrong with me because I wasn't sleeping at all. And they moved me out to Male Three the next day. Oakley.[1] It was maximum security. Forensic. It was Auckland's Lake Alice.[2]

The day room I was released into was ninety feet by forty feet, and there were ninety criminals in the room. Savage, the superintendent, had this policy of taking anybody from Paremoremo that threatened to slash their wrists. There were about two or three psychotic patients and the rest of them were criminals. They had all the chairs around the walls. I had to stand in the centre of the room. I was smashed in the face many times by criminals. I was psychotic, and I was left psychotic for a month under observation. I mean, I didn't sleep all that time. I went a month without sleep. Then they gave me fluphenazine, which really knocked the hell out of me. It was a very bad drug for me, and I was taken before the Court and I was given a 39J – criminally insane.[3]

So here began a five-year saga in Male Three.[4] Three months, even if you got really well in a hurry. You'd spend three months in lock-up. Three months in the open ward, and then you would be discharged into a boarding house.

I did that many times because initially I was on fluphenazine, then

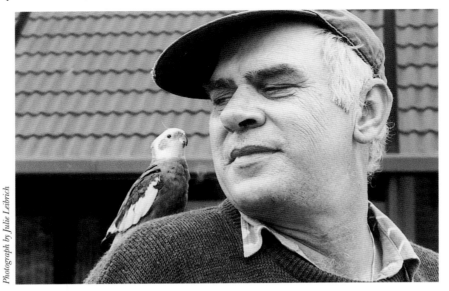

Photograph by Julie Leibrich

depixol, then lithium, and every time I got high again. I'd go out and I would say, this mania is never going to happen again. You know, I'd be as well in the remission as I am here today, and I'd think to myself that this is never going to happen again and I'm going to take all sorts of precautions. I'll take that lithium until I'm blue in the face. I'm going to get on top of this illness. I'm going to put it behind me. I got various jobs as a tool-maker, as a pattern-maker. I'd be out in the community for about three or four months, up to six months, and then all of a sudden the mania would start to happen again.

In the five years that I was in Male Three I went through 22,000 locked doors. Every door I went through was locked. I mean your cell door was locked. The door up to the stairs to the cell rooms was locked, the door at the bottom of the stairs was locked. The tea room door was locked. The day room door was locked. The kitchen door was locked. The dining room door was locked. Every door you went through was unlocked before you and locked after you. I went through 22,000 locked doors.

Very few people visited me in Oakley, because they never thought I would get out and I was just a nutter. It hurt. But in a way, it's just par for the course, you know; it's just they don't understand.

I had about seven or eight re-admissions. I would turn up at the hospital at the weekend saying, *I am going high.* I knew I had about a day's warning in those days. I'd turn up on the weekend and say, *I'm going high.* They'd

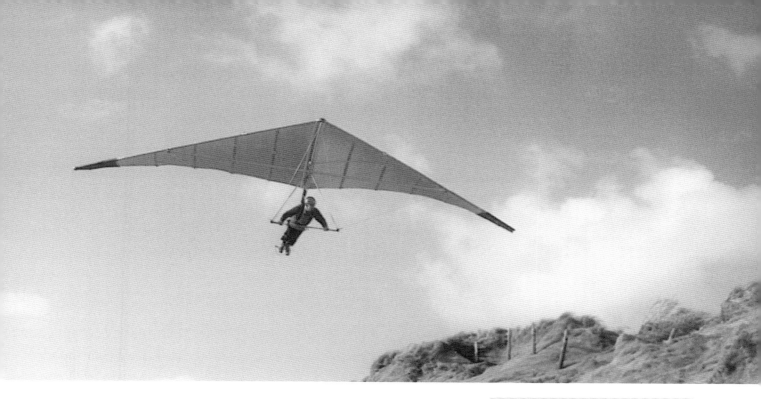

say, *Don't bother us, it's the weekend, come back and see us on Monday.*

Well, by Monday I'd gone and stayed at the Sheraton Hotel without money, or invaded a Control Tower …

One time at the airport I jumped a six-foot fence, and then ran up the stairs, all the way up to the top of the control tower. Nowadays there is a huge fence around the tower. A friend of mine was in a plane taxiing into Auckland, and the passenger in the next seat said, *Look at that fence that they've built around that control tower – that's huge, that's massive, it's very high.* And he said, *Yes, and I know the man who was responsible for having that built!*

It was the energy that would start building up in my system, and I wouldn't sleep. I would go a night without sleep, and then if I went another night without sleep I knew I was in trouble. I would go and try and get help, and then I would lose the insight. Two or three days later I would lose the insight. If they didn't catch me in the first day when I was compliant with their regime, then I didn't want to know about the system, and I'd play merry hell.

Finally, in 1984, having been in hospital four years, off and on, I decided that I was going to start a chart. I tried to prove that lithium wasn't an effective medication, and that I was going high despite taking it. In a hos-

Alasdair hang gliding. 'In 1973 I saw a photo of a hang glider, well right from the start I wanted a company making hang gliders, so I went to America, got a couple of trips, teamed up with a partner, and we started a company called Pacific Kites.'

pital environment, the medication just wasn't working.

They wouldn't comply with that chart, you know. When my moods started to rise, they wouldn't fill the chart out. They said I was just too stroppy. So I said to them, *Right, I'm not going to take your medication any more, I'm not going to take it.*

I went through from April '84 until about August without the drug. I just had cycles of deep depression and elation, deep depression and elation, really oscillating mood, rapid cycling of mood, fast cycling of mood. But then, on my birthday, the hour I turned thirty-three (at ten o'clock, the hour I was born) I had an out-of-body experience where I left my body for two weeks. I can remember bubbling up from the bottom of my feet, boiling up out of my body and another spirit coming into this body and looking after it for two weeks. I can remember the spot where I re-entered my body two weeks later.

While I was away, this body had stars in its head. I can remember leaving the earth, the earth and the moon, the earth and the moon and the sun, our galaxy. And I just kept going out and out and out and out. Basically my body had become impossible to inhabit. I'd purged myself, I had abandoned everything, I was leaving, I'd gone. And the return was incredibly difficult. I chose to come back for some reason, to complete something. I was going to return through the universe back into this body that I'd left in Male Three, and I remember the moment that I came back into the body. I was sitting in a chair, and all of a sudden … The interesting thing was that when I came back into my body I had to steady myself. I couldn't stand up, because of the earth's rotation. I could feel the earth rotating.

While I was away, somebody gave the body haloperidol which meant that I had to return, which was hell. It brought my body under control to the point that I could now return to it.

In retrospect, I cannot understand for the life of me why it took them five years to use what they should have used in the first month of my admission, which was haloperidol. It's an anti-manic, antipsychotic. I had tried other medications. I was initially tried on lithium, and then when I was in Oakley I was tried on fluphenazine, depixol, tegretol, lithium, chlorpromazine. I've been on virtually the whole range of them, but never in the five years did they try haloperidol – never.

In fact, in 1983, while I was still in hospital, I got a message through to an airline pilot doctor and asked him specifically was there an anti-psychotic tranquilliser that would give me protection from highs. And he came back and said, *Yes there is, go and see your psychiatrist.* I went to Savage and asked him. All he said was, *You may not be sensitive to lithium carbonate,* end of story. He didn't pursue the matter any further and I spent a further two years in hospital.

I think that without any form of medication the mind went so manic that I simply couldn't inhabit the body any more, and some spirit was able to look after my body while I was gone. I mean, in the olden days, manics died of exhaustion, and I think that's what happened to me. I exhausted myself and I left my body, and there was some spirit there that said, *He's not ready to go yet, we'll look after this body and he'll return.* Because when I left, as I was leaving, a voice, which I produced, this body produced, but coming from the spirit said, *It's all right, we've got him now.* I was protected.

There's a saying that keeps me going, by Meher Baba,[5] which means compassionate father in Indian, and it's something I saw about ten years ago. I liked it so much I memorised it. It goes something like this:

> To penetrate into the essence of all being and significance, and release the fragrance of that inner attainment for the guidance and benefit of others by expressing in the world of form love, truth, beauty and purity. This is the sole gain that has any intrinsic and absolute worth. All other happenings and incidents in themselves can have no lasting importance.

That's what keeps me going.

Meher Baba. It's in my mind all the time. It's as vivid as my drive from that car park to here this afternoon. It's with me all the time. I know what happened to me. It's subjective, I can't express it in any other way. I know that people have had these experiences. Before that experience, if anyone had said to me they had an out-of-body experience like that, I would have dismissed it with a grain of salt. But, you know, it's happened to me. The results speak for themselves, ten years of good health.

Basically the madness stopped in '84. I've been off all sections for nine years.[6] I'm on the invalid's benefit now. I'd been on a sickness benefit and working, you know, six months here, six months there full-time. After you've been psychotic, you're never the same. Your tolerance to people, especially in an employer-employee relationship, wears thin after a while, and I just couldn't tolerate it. After coming out of the aircraft industry and being highly trained in very meticulous repair work, to go back into common industry – it's just not the same cup of tea. You just can't achieve the same standards.

Now I go to a GP for my medication. Every three months I pick up

Opposite: Alasdair's
Engineering Trade certificate

Motley and Jessie. 'I built a
perch for Jessie, a pedestal,
and I got him out of his cage
and he was sitting on his
pedestal and he could fly, his
wings, his wings had grown
back and he could fly.'

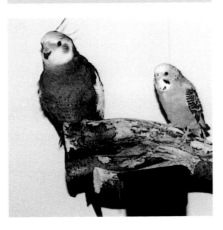

another three months' supply. I have no psychiatrist. This recovery was done without counselling, was done without a psychiatrist. It was just haloperidol. That was all I required. And to think they locked me up for five years on all sorts of medications except haloperidol, only for somebody to try it at the end – somebody who wasn't part of the hospital system.

To start with, I had a very materialistic view of life. I thought that money was the thing that I should pursue, and that all other things would come with money. But I have learnt that it's values and insight and wisdom, and keeping true to yourself, having a conviction that's with you as a strength that you can fall back on.

My needs are met. My mother has provided me with a home unit and a car, because I keep my relationship with my mother and my family in good standing now. I keep in touch with my brothers overseas. I keep in touch with my family. Through that, I've regained my place, my role in life.

I live on my own. I've had to learn to overcome loneliness. The secret, one of the secrets to living alone, is to have something – it may be a plant, it may be a pet, a bird, a cat, a dog – but get something that you have to care for outside of yourself. Because by caring for something else it also helps you care about yourself. By taking an interest in something outside of yourself, it makes you look after yourself. I've had a cockatiel for nine years, and he's taught me a lot. I had two, I had Jessie, then Motley. You know, that cockatiel, if I leave his cage open (he's got a large cage), in the morning I'll find him on my shoulder. His wings are clipped, he can't fly. He's made his way out of the cage, down off the table, onto the carpet, across the floor, up onto the bed, onto my shoulder and that's where he sits, because he cares about me. He's got a travelling cage at the moment with me at the motel, but when he's at home he sits in a cathedral.

Pets will reward you in so many ways, you know. The last bird I had, Jessie, I remember coming home one night, a bit under the weather, and this bird – I built a perch for him, a pedestal – and I got him out of his cage and he was sitting on his pedestal and he could fly. His wings had grown back and he could fly. Well, I went in and crashed on my bed. He saw me and flew into my room after I was lying in my bed, paralysed. I was really depressed. He flew in, landed on my pillow, gave me a kiss on the lips, and then flew back to his perch, and then three minutes later he was back again giving me another kiss. They are very sensitive birds.

People ask me where I get my support from. What's happened is, through my recovery on haloperidol, I've been able to restore all my relationships with people – people that didn't want to know me when I was ill, never visited me. I've reconnected with those people, and they form a network of about 400 that I communicate with over any one month. That's where my support comes from – from those people that have seen me well, seen me ill, and then see me recovered.

I worked for six years, I delivered the local rag to New Lynn township. I walked 500 miles a year for six years. That's 3,000 miles in a circle around New Lynn township, three times a week. But I've stopped that, and I've also stopped a cleaning job to devote more time to mental health issues. I want to become a consumer consultant with the Mason Clinic, because I think I've got a great story, and I can be a great advocate for mental health and people that have recovered on medication.

Over the last year I've set up the Manic Depression Information Trust in Auckland. I wrote a submission to the Mason Inquiry.[7] I wanted to see a mood disorder clinic in Auckland, specialising just in that field, so if people require acute services there would be a specialist mood disorder clinic. Because, you see, the intellect is left unaffected with a mood disorder, and that's the thing. We're not disabled in any other way, but we've got a racing mind that no one can handle.

Very few people can avoid life without some kind of medication,

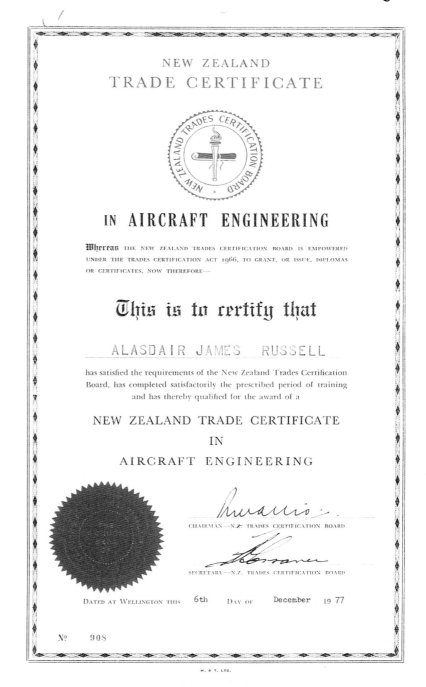

whether it be lithium, or lithium and tegretol and chlorpromazine (or in my case haloperidol). I'm not saying we should put haloperidol in the water supply or anything like that, but I think very few who suffer from a mood disorder can cure it or control it without medication. I don't know many.

You have to protect your affect.[8] Look after your mood, because if you don't, it will kill you. If you don't look after that mood of yours, if it gets too low …

I monitor my moods on a scale of zero to a hundred. At a hundred you are God, at fifty you are normal, and at zero God doesn't exist. I've been all three. And I know what one I would prefer to be. I would prefer to be God, but no one could handle me.

I know my moods, I know that I am probably sixty, sixty-five this after-

Alasdair's obituary from the Western Leader, Thursday, 5 March 1998.

Alasdair fought to overcome barriers

OBITUARY

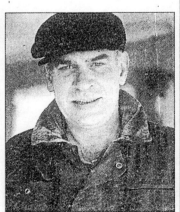

ALASDAIR RUSSELL

New Lynn has lost one of its local identities.

Alasdair Russell has died aged 43, but will be long remembered by New Lynn retailers who came to know him well during his thrice weekly visits to deliver the *Western Leader*.

Mr Russell loved his delivery job and often quipped that it gave him 300 instant friends.

New Lynn retailer Julie Halligan says Mr Russell was a real personality in the New Lynn area.

"He was a really lovely guy and a really interesting and intelligent guy. He would always stop in for a chat and he will be sorely missed," Ms Halligan says.

Mr Russell, a long-time suffer of manic depression, was also well known in west Auckland for his commitment to improve the lives of other sufferers of manic depression.

In the months before his death, Mr Russell was devoted to setting up the West Auckland Manic Depression Information Trust.

"He wanted to destigmatise the issue and he knew first hand about it. He wanted to provide more information about the disease for people suffering, those close to them and the general public," says friend Jim Gladwin.

Mr Gladwin says Mr Russell was a compassionate man who fought hard to overcome the barriers of manic depression.

Mr Russell also had an interest in flying and was involved in some of this country's first glider flights.

"He did not have many worldly means, but he gave of his time freely. He was a bright, intelligent man who was handicapped by this illness, but managed to battle against it," Mr Gladwin says.

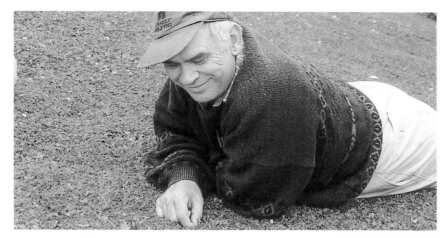

noon, and I'll have to take some haloperidol. Tonight I'll sleep and tomorrow I'll be fifty again, I'll come down. The depression, I'm always working on that, I'm always treating myself to something, giving myself little rewards. It may be an extra shave a day. It may be an ice-cream as you're passing the shop. Just treating yourself to something each day to make life a little bit more pleasurable. It's a normal mood that you've got to protect, and if it sinks and you're not looking after yourself, well ...

I've started to collect names of people with manic depression. I've got sixty names now. In the back of the book I've started to keep a list of people that have died through manic depression, through depression caused by manic depression. I've got fourteen names there. Twenty per cent of the people who suffer from manic depression will successfully kill themselves – twenty per cent.

So if I have a worry at the moment, it's how I am going to look after my mood, how I'm going to protect myself.

Postscript

Alasdair died on 13 February 1998. Despite all his bravery and courage, he was finally one of the twenty per cent who did not survive.

I met his mother, Jeannie Wilson, in the last week of preparing this book for the publisher. We talked about Alasdair's story and his life and we chose these pictures of Alasdair together.

Discovering the life you want, says

Julie Leibrich

Julie is fifty-one and a Mental Health Commissioner. She has worked for twenty years as a social scientist and is a registered psychologist. She is also a poet and writer of children's stories and lives on the Kapiti Coast.

My life has been enormously influenced by episodes of depression. They took away years of my life as a young woman. They influenced the *path* of my life for twenty years. They were the reason I didn't have a family until it was too late to do so. I lost homes. I lost a husband. I lost friends. I lost many things I otherwise might have had. I almost lost my life. Now, the episodes are less frequent and I have much more ability to deal with them.

I can remember being depressed when I was quite young and then it got to quite serious proportions when I was a student at Edinburgh University. I was sent to see a psychiatrist, but he was a bit too keen to slap a label on me and I didn't like that. He said I was 'pre-schizophrenic' and had to go into hospital. But I refused. For a long time after that I avoided anything that smacked of medical intervention.

Over the next few years I had several episodes of depression but managed to cope. Looking back, life seemed pretty bleak a lot of the time. I was in a very lonely sort of marriage and we moved around different countries. So I never felt settled and never really made lasting friends.

I came to New Zealand when I was twenty-seven and took a second degree, in psychology. But during those years my depression worsened and I had to look for help again. Even the littlest things were very difficult for me to do. I was supposed to be embarking on a PhD, yet I felt my brain was like porridge.

Nothing seemed to help. Then a friend of mine died in a horrific car accident and while I was on my way back from a trip to Britain, my father, whom I loved very much, died and I wasn't there at the time. I was on the other side of the world.

I went into a kind of dead state for about a year. I don't really remember anything else from that year. I don't really remember the rest of the year. It's like it isn't there any more.

Looking back now, I think that I was terribly drugged out for most of the time. For about three years I was on various antidepressants and later, after I saw a psychiatrist, I was on more and heavier drugs – major tranquillisers and anti-psychotics. I was like a walking cocktail. It was horrendous.

I was pre-occupied with killing myself. That went on for months but eventually the thoughts became much more specific and finally I started to plan my death. I was also having hallucinations at times, and was admitted to a psychiatric hospital early in 1979.

I thought I'd gone to hell. I hated it. I hated all the drugs. I think that experience more than any other took away my self-esteem. But it was in that context that I met the person who finally saved me, in a way. I had a wonderful therapist who was prepared to come inside to the world I was living in, rather than trying to get me to come out into theirs. It meant I wasn't alone with my terror. And I could begin to deal with it.

But I was seen as a bit of a troublemaker at that hospital, because I pushed for patients' rights. I have told this story elsewhere and it is too long to tell here.[1] But the result was that I was put in isolation and threatened with ECT. When I think about it now, I see myself in that room coming to a very profound decision that day. It was that I would lie. I would do anything it took to act like 'normal people' acted so that I could get out.

After I got out things got even worse. While I was in hospital, my husband told me he had begun an affair, and shortly after I got home he went to live with her. So now I was alone in the house that had once been ours. I was still terribly depressed and found it very frightening. I used to hear noises and voices at night. One night I tried to commit suicide. It was the only attempt I ever made and I stuffed it up. I took some pills but vomited and so I survived. But I just wanted to die.

The next thing, I am in a psychiatric unit. I don't remember a lot. It's like looking back and seeing three or four frames of an entire film. And one of the frames I see is being force fed chlorpromazine. I remember pushing this nurse's hand away and saying, *I don't want any more.* I remember them forcing the syrup down my throat. It's probably one of my worst memories.

I've got those frames and I can also see the space in the ward door when I finally left. I can see the gap between the two doors. The way they opened. I remember that.

I eventually managed to talk my way out of hospital. I just knew I had to leave that place and it seemed to me crucial that I left before the New Year began, before midnight.

I said I wanted to discharge myself and I was told that I wasn't well enough to do so. But I insisted. Thank God the doctor I spoke to accepted that, but he also warned me that if there were problems, I could very easily be committed now. I was filled with terror about that for a long time.

But it was a wonderful thing for me not to take their advice, to disregard it. That was the turning-point in my life. That was the beginning of the person I became.

I remember that first night out terribly clearly, writing the New Year in, in a journal. I wrote right through the hour of midnight. It was the beginning of a new decade. I had lost almost everything. My marriage. My home. Some friends. The community I had lived in. My future. And there was an enormous resolve in me that night that I would survive.

I think the last twenty years has been a slow, slow learning process. I

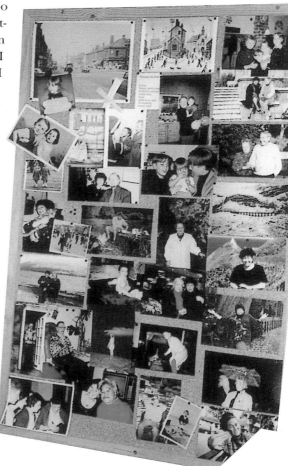

Far away family and friends.

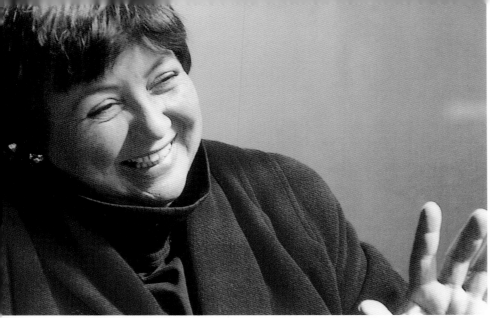

Photograph by Roger Hewitson

didn't want to live until a few years ago. So my actions were mostly about escape. It wasn't about recovery at all. It's only in the last few years that I have begun to recover. For several years I actively wanted to die and most of my energy was spent in trying to not achieve that. Then I returned to a phase where I didn't mind if I died, and even hoped I would, from the age of about thirty-three to forty-three. Then I realised I actively wanted to live. And that was the next turning-point.

I'd been working on a book called *Straight to the Point* and been interviewing people about why they had given up crime or at least given up *most* crime. That was a profound experience for me, doing that book.[2] I loved that book. I think it was my first true act of creation as a writer. I gave it everything I had. And I felt that I had really created a piece of literature as well as research.

People talked about the turning-points in their life. They told me what it was which made them realise life had value. And that's what affected me, because as I interviewed and spent time with these people, it made me ask myself, *What value does life have for me?*

Towards the very end of writing that book I was walking on the beach one day and I remember having a sort of vision, really. I looked back over my shoulder down the beach towards Pukerua Bay and I saw a long line and at the end it was me at eighty. So I saw myself at eighty on the beach, backwards.

I looked at this me and said, *You can't wait for me any longer, I'll come now.* So what I'm trying to say is that I looked at me at eighty and I knew for the first time I couldn't wait any longer to be me. I couldn't wait. I had to start being me. That was a profound realisation.

It had a quality about it of a revelation. That's all, it had some strange quality. I knew then that I was a writer. I had always said to myself that I'd wait until I retired to do the things I wanted to do. So from that point on I could see some point in living because I could see these things that I wanted to do *now*.

I got home, put a pen in my hand and started writing. Since then one of the most important things in my life is writing. I love words. I love language. I'll never stop because *I am* a writer. I knew that before, but it took me years to start writing.

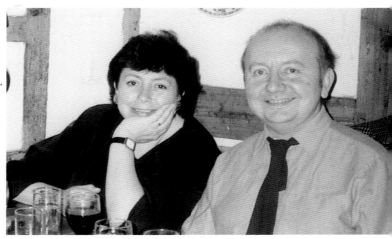

Me with my brother Tony.

The other thing was to learn to live alone. To live alone was a necessity at that time in my life. To learn to live alone was a bonus. Bit by bit I conquered fears that I had about it. Classic fear being the Friday night when you think everybody's married, happy, and having a great time downtown. I learned to value just being on my own. I'm alone a lot but I don't often feel lonely. I think it's because I'm with myself. And I love my home. To me, my home is a haven, a very very safe place. I bought this home seven years ago. And it's by the sea, which is terribly meaningful to me. I just love being at home.

There are certain cornerstones to my staying well. To be me is the biggest cornerstone. I have quite a history of leaving my body, leaving myself, 'disappearing'. And making other people 'disappear'. Doing a kind of psychic escape. I have to stay *within* myself. Despite everything, to stay *with* myself.

Friends are another. I have some wonderful friends – friends who inspire me and amaze me really. And I'm so grateful that they put up with me! I'm not an easy friend. I'm a *good* friend, but not an *easy* friend because I set limits on what I can do. I can't afford to be around people who need more of me than I can give, because it's in my nature to try and meet the need and I get emotionally bankrupt too easily. So I have to have friends who understand that I am quite limited in some ways, and that I like enormous amounts of time on my own.

A sense of belonging is another cornerstone. I have spent much of my life feeling like an alien. I felt I never belonged anywhere. Or with anybody. I was always outside looking in, or inside looking out. I was never in the present, always in the past or the future. Now I belong – in this community, in a circle of friends, in a group of family, in a group of colleagues. I belong on this beach by this sea. I belong in this house. That's because this is where I *want* to be. And I belong to me because I'm *who* I want to be.

One of the other cornerstones which has been crucial has been the right help at the right time – drugs and counselling. The judicious use of drugs, and the judicious *non*-use of drugs. Ironically, I had refused to take medication for about seventeen years, then shortly after I was asked to become a Mental Health Commissioner, several very stressful things happened in my life. The same week I accepted this job and new and demanding role, Doug, my second husband, had a heart attack. Within the next month, I was admitted to hospital myself with a physical crisis and shortly after I got home, there was a fire on my property. I started to spiral down in a way I couldn't control and for the first time in all those years, with the help of my GP, *chose* to use medication as one of my tools. I found that quite liberating. In a way, I conquered another fear.

I have also used counselling, very very good counselling. As a psychologist, I have a supervisor with whom I can discuss difficult work issues. She is also is a counsellor for me and is absolutely superb. She has a very light touch and it's spot on! Sometimes she has helped me do some crucial psycho-dynamic work, which has advanced my psychological development by many years.[3]

I believe there are points of readiness for psychological development – points of readiness for maturity. I now believe that time has a job to do and I have to let it do it. That's been a very significant recognition for me. That there are some things only time can do. It's to do with readiness.

I also think that we should be able to forget. We should allow time to let us forget the things which have caused too much pain. I kept a detailed journal during the worst years of being depressed, and one day decided to burn it, because there were some things I *wanted* to forget. I've never regretted that.

There's one thing I know I've not really sorted out yet. For most of my life I've had only two gears, top gear and reverse, and I've never noticed any other gears in between. My working pattern in a period of creativity, for instance. I can go for three or four days without sleep, and have done, but it's not a sensible thing to do at my age. It's been suggested that these are 'manic episodes'. However I know that for me that pattern indicates a period of enormous creativity. And I know that by experience.

It's been crucial for me to make the distinction between medical categorisation and human experience. I've been very fortunate in having highs, and they are tied to periods of creativity. But I have to manage them, because if I don't, I spin out too far and too fast. I have to impose balance in my life, but I haven't learnt to manage that as well as I'd like. That is an area of potential development, you might say!

If anybody is ever going to diagnose me, it's going to be me. And I choose not to diagnose myself because I don't yet understand the connection between physiological change, intellectual change, life events, nature, nurture, environment, and a spiritual life. And I don't think *they* do.

It's not *the* illness I need to know about, it's *my* illness. That's what I need to know, not just what it says in the textbook or what someone else tells me. What is *my* version like? How does it affect me? How do I predict it? How do I know when the earthquake's coming? What are the tremors that come before? And what do I do when the birds stop singing? Well, I try to do something *before* the birds stop singing.

I've really come to understand how to look after my mental health, even though I don't always do it. I've finally worked out what I need to do to prevent severe depression. I also have a kind of tool-kit which I can use if my depression gets too severe despite my attempts at prevention. Again, I've written about this before.[4] But there are some things I really need to mention.

The first is touch. I've got to ask for touch. After touch, sound is the next sense. I don't go a day without music. Music is crucial. I use it as some people use pills – to modify my emotions. I couldn't bear a world without music.

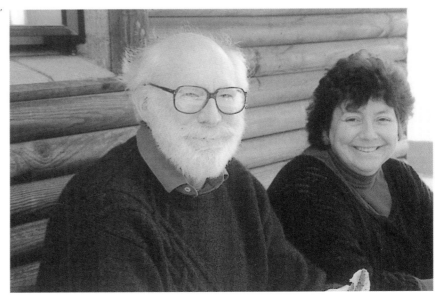

Doug and me.

I remember years of not seeing colour. I mean, to me colour now is one of the most wonderful things in the world. I remember not tasting things, not seeing things, not hearing things. Not feeling touch. Loss of life's feeling is one of the worst aspects of depression for me.

I also believe in the great 'as if'. Even when I'm extremely depressed it is helpful to act as if I am not. It's not about denying that I

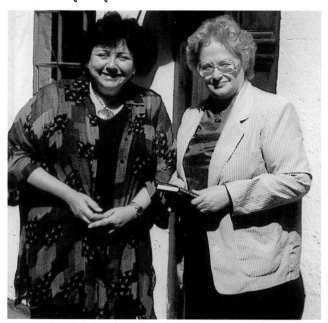

Betty and me.

Opposite: Covers of three of my books:
The Paper Road. (Steele Roberts, 1998.)
Straight to the Point: Angles on Giving up Crime. (Otago University Press, 1993.)
The Ossossossorus. (Scholastic New Zealnd, 1999.)

am depressed, it's about acting *as if* I'm not. It makes a difference.

Some people get their energy from other people. I don't. I nearly always get my energy from myself. But when I'm under the dark spell, I sometimes need people to remind me that I can be different. I sometimes need people to help me reverse the spell. There are very few people I've met who can do that, but there *are* some. What is special about them for me? I suppose I see them as soul-mates.

What are we once we've stripped away everything? I've had to learn that when everything else is gone, there is still something there. That's the space within the heart, and that's where I can be when everything is stripped away.[5] And I have to keep that space safe no matter what.

So I also have to look after myself spiritually. That's another cornerstone. I have to feed my soul, because once I stop doing that, then I may no longer be available to myself as a safe place. And I feed my soul with poetry, music, nature, silence and solitude.

I intend to be a wise old woman by the time I'm eighty-one, and I won't have disappeared off that beach. I'll still be there.

Postscript

When I began this book, about two years ago, it was because I wanted to contribute something positive to the images we have of people with a mental illness. I also wanted more insight into how to deal successfully with mental illness.

I started simply by thinking about recovery, asking myself what does it involve? What will people say about it? What does it mean to 'recover'? However as I listened to people, I began to struggle with the word 'recovery'. Some people in the book were quite comfortable with the word, and talked about stages of recovery. Others didn't want to use the word, because it can imply a simple and finite solution. Yet very few of us had a story which said, *This happened and I got over it and I'm a box of birds now.* In fact, I don't think *any* of us said that.

Most of the stories I heard were about serious and life-changing illness, and perhaps that is why I am so struck by the complexity of the process of getting well. As people talked about dealing with illness, their stories were about the progressive discovery of solutions.

At the same time, something else emerged, something more expansive than discovering how to deal with illness. People talked about the discoveries they had made about themselves. I have often felt that dealing with my own illness has given me something beyond recovery, something more than recovery. And now I heard others say the same. This was a precious insight.

So, at this point in my understanding (when I have to overcome my fear of the permanence of publication), if there were one word I would choose to describe what I heard throughout this work, it would be **DISCOVERY**. The stories told to me were full of discovery – not just *about* dealing with mental illness but *through* dealing with it.

Right now, the best way I can describe dealing with mental illness is **making our way along an ever-widening spiral of discovery** in which we uncover problems, discover the best ways to deal with them, recover ground that has been lost, discover new things about ourselves, then uncover deeper problems, discover the best ways… and so on in an intricate process of growth.

I think that most people, at least in the world I know, attempt to make sense of their lives, and when a profound experience (such as a mental illness) strikes us, we struggle to make sense of that too. Why did it happen? What caused it? We may even impose an explanation. But sometimes there *is* no meaning – at least not one we understand. Then we have to put up with the pain of not understanding and eventually we have to *put aside the need to know.*

What I began to understand through listening to the others' stories and thinking about my own was that getting well and staying well depend on coming to terms with meaning. Ultimately, we are able *either* to make sense of things *or* to accept that we cannot. I think this is a very important point because it is to do with getting peace of mind. It means we can stop asking, Why *did this happen?* and start asking, How *can I best deal with this experience?*

I also saw that, at some point, people began to take control of the things that were in their power to control, and through this, they began to get well. What is so poignant for me about this realisation is that I think we still have a mental health system which is built on a model of controlling people. Perhaps this is why the decision to take charge so often rises up from an experience of bad treatment – as if a person is finally forced to say, *I'm going to find my own way through this.*

People told me about some disgraceful things which happened to them while they were in mental health services. And I once experienced them

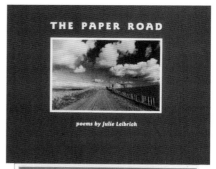

THE PAPER ROAD

poems by Julie Leibrich

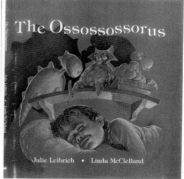

The Ossossossorus

Julie Leibrich • Linda McClelland

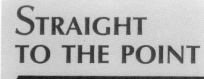

STRAIGHT TO THE POINT

Angles on Giving Up Crime

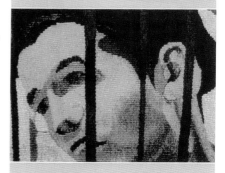

Julie Leibrich

myself. Some of them do not even appear in this book because of the shame some of us feel about having 'allowed' ourselves to be treated in this way. At times, as a Mental Health Commissioner, I felt ashamed to be connected with the system. Even though these accounts were about historical events, I am aware that some of the things people talked about still happen and that the treatment can be far worse than the condition.

It is also so clear to me what a wonderful difference it makes when you meet a really good health professional, whether it is a nurse, psychiatrist, counsellor, GP, social worker, key-worker, or whatever. But what is the essence of 'really good'? It's not just having knowledge and skills, it's using them with *respect* for the person you are treating. The therapist might be the expert on the illness, but the person is the expert on themselves. A partnership of *real* power!

I think it is about the nature of *relationship*. It is to do with giving someone the chance to say what is going on for them and actually listening. Seeing, if you like, 'their side of the story'. This came across to me, for instance, as I listened to what people said about their experiences with medication. It can take a long time to accept that you need and are willing to take drugs, especially when you have had some dreadful experiences with medication. It's only when you find someone who actually listens to those experiences, and helps you sort out the best drug and right dosage, that drugs can do their job.

On a deeper level, the 'therapeutic relationship' also depends on making it possible actually to relate. When I gathered these stories, I did not set out on a path of healing. Yet a lot of people said that the *process* of telling their story to me was healing for them. There were times of laughter and fun in almost every interview, but there were lots of tears as well. Almost every person in the book cried at some point when they were telling their story – and it was not just the pain of the memories, it was also a kind of relief in sharing them.

The experience was healing for me too. I was always touched in some way by a person's story. This morning, as I write, I still feel very moved by the whole process. I am deeply aware of the pain that we have suffered because of mental illness. Yet through that pain, and often anger, came the determination to survive. But we have to survive not only the illness, but also the consequences of it – the lost things that we may never recover. And finally, we have to survive the memories. That is why it is so terribly important that we can also see what we have gained from the experience. And that others recognise that, too.

I believe that people heal themselves. I say this because I see treatment as something that happens from outside, whereas healing happens from within. This is why I believe that the voice inside, which tells a person what they need, should be listened to. I heard about many different kinds of treatment, from traditional to new age, from sophisticated to simple, but what I heard most of all was that we got well when we found the treatment which was *right for us* (and rejected the ones which were not). That is to say, we make wise choices, based on our expert knowledge of ourselves. And that is why we need a range of choices in health care.

I also saw people make wise choices about 'expert' opinion on them. The people in these stories *questioned* things – we didn't just accept what we were told. And I think this is one of the reasons why we got well.

Diagnosis is usually determined by someone else, standing outside the person – someone else tells you what's 'wrong' with you. And diagnosis usually comes along with a prognosis attached to it – someone else tells you what the outcome is likely to be. But if all you have is someone else's diagnosis and prognosis, then your recovery might also be prescribed by that. That is to say, someone else will tell you when you are 'right'.

Looking closely at what people said, many of us had to question our diagnosis and prognosis *in order* to get well. I think this is terribly important to understand because our stories all showed that **recovery is self-defined**. It is defined, in fact, through **discovery**.

Diagnosis is a rather subjective science and one which is still evolving. In these stories, we talked about the need to understand our 'diagnosis'. But we weren't talking about text books – we were talking about insight into our own experience.

Insight is one of the most wonderful things we have, as human beings. It is the thing which takes us beyond information and knowledge. It is the key to wisdom. I think information is just about facts – things that are usually told to us. Knowledge comes from integrating those facts. But wisdom comes through understanding – standing *under* knowledge and allowing the insight we gain from our own experience to illuminate knowledge. That is what is in these stories – wisdom. And that's why they are so valuable. That's why you need to hear them.

For instance, I see wisdom in the way many of us interpreted diagnosis in terms of vulnerability. This meant we could see how to protect ourselves better, and begin a kind of practice of natural prevention. I am talking here about the ordinary things people tend to do when they have a good life. I mean the things some of you may take for granted – like being kind to yourself, getting enough rest, some exercise, eating nutritious food, having little treats, having fun. What is extraordinary is that for many of us with a mental illness, seeing the importance of these things is a kind of revelation. They are something we have to *learn* how to do, and then do almost self-consciously, until they become second nature.

Then, of course, there are the 'bigger things' to do with finding your place in the world – a home, family, friends, loving relationships, people who know and value you for who you are (not for who you might become), a sense of belonging, a sense of purpose, feeling useful. You might say, well of course! But these are the very things which are so often denied to those of us with a mental illness *because* of the illness. Yet when doors are opened and we are able to take our place in the world it makes all the difference to dealing with mental illness.

People need their place in the world, not just a place in hospital, or on a 'case-load'. For me, this is one of the strongest arguments of all for the closure of large 'warehouse' psychiatric hospitals. The trouble is that *community-based* care came to be understood as being *community* care. And we all know what happens when *that* doesn't work – when the community *doesn't* care, or when it doesn't *want* to care, when it doesn't know *how* to care, or when it isn't funded well enough to be able to care. 'Out in the community' is a very cold abstract term, in these circumstances. But what *is* a community, anyway?

It's easy to see what a community is in traditional terms, in the sense of a small village, or an extended family, or a small local neighbourhood. But is there really such a thing as a community in the centre of a big city? Or a whole country? I think not, at least not in the sense of shared interests and meaningful relationships.

In the mental health system, we need to clarify our concept of community, if community-based care is really going to work. *Community* needs to be understood as something much smaller, if community-based care is to make real sense. What I heard people talk about was their warm and intimate worlds – family, whanau, circle of friends, workplace, local neighbourhood, their small town.

Finally, there is spirituality. I think talking about personal spirituality is one of the hardest things to do in our society. And because we are not accustomed to talking about it easily, we are losing the words. It's like the last bastion of silence – after sex, politics and money. Talking about spirituality often seems to cheapen it, and embarrasses some people. In the absence of shared meaning in words, there is sometimes a sense of hollowness or pretentiousness when people talk about 'being spiritual'. But without a doubt, what I heard people talk about was the importance of spiritual ease.

Coming to terms with the knowledge that you *have* a mental illness is almost as difficult a personal task as coming to terms with the illness itself. What does it mean to come to terms with it? I think it means acceptance. Seeing it as being only *a part* of who you are. Learning to live with it, staying real and honest about it, and having an environment which makes this possible.

Just because you *have* an illness does not mean you are always ill. And one of the hardest parts of accepting the illness is accepting that you *might* get ill again – the symptoms might recur. This may be true of learning to deal with any serious illness, but with mental illness I think there is the added barb of 'internalised discrimination'. If we get ill again, we often feel worthless again, even though we have once said to ourselves *This is the score.* The insights of self-acceptance which we have when we are well are hard to hold on to when we are ill. This is why it is crucial to have people who believe in us and give us hope.

Again and again, I heard about the benefits that illness brought: how the very experience made people stronger, and how the courage they found to deal with the illness meant they achieved things they had never thought possible. I think this is why some of us say that mental illness is a gift – because you can discover many wonderful things about yourself **through** dealing with it.

This is not in any way to deny the suffering involved. In fact, I think it's the very process of dealing with that suffering which brings one of its greatest gifts – strength of character. I suppose this is true of overcoming any adversity in life generally, but I think those of us with mental illness are tested in ways which are sometimes unimaginable to others. Partly, this is because mental anguish is often invisible, and partly because we are often forced to conceal it from others. Perhaps that is one of the reasons why there is so little recognition of the heroic journeys of discovery that we have to make. And why prejudice against us is so particularly cruel.

One of the most distressing things about mental illness is that it often involves a disintegration of self. So dealing with it, and surviving it, almost inevitably means that there has to be some kind of reintegration of one's self. This 'putting yourself back together' can lead to valuing things about yourself which you may never have even recognised before.

You can come to see, for instance, that the very same sensitivity which at

THE ICE MAIDEN

On the steppes of Russia, my threshold
was finally found. A long incoming
to enchantment. It was not until
the dawn stroked my face
after these lost years of icy
lamentation, that I opened my eyes
and let the day come in.

The workmen at the site were startled
to see my warm tears flow. Could not
explain away the fire field in their view
or the way their hands were warmed
on touching me.

Silent I lay amidst my treasures
for they had carpeted my tomb with silk
and sacrificed six horses to lie with me.
Cold company at night. No light
from those eyes.

No dreamers there. Only I knew
the years of solitude. Yet never spoke
of it, nor gave a sign of my entrapment
here. Myself included in deceit
I did not know my state of frozen grief

until the sun came in
then
amazed.

Julie Leibrich

Ice Maiden Melts After 2,500 Years
She wore a long white dress with two red stripes, a matching
blouse and spectacular head-dress Her ears were adorned with
gold her arms and hands bore tattoos of mythical monsters. She
lay on her side, her head to the east in the hollowed lidded trunk
of a larch tree decorated with carvings of geese and snow
leopards. Natasha Polosmak the Russian archaeologist who
discovered her had never seen anything like it.
Star-Times, April 1994.

times is the dark side of the illness also brings light, and means you can have something very precious to give to the world – a deep capacity for compassion. And the closeness to a sense of dying, which some mental illnesses bring, can create a profound appreciation of life. Also, for some people, the dividing line between creativity and 'madness' is very fine and the link between highs and creativity is as clear as day.

You also come to see that, at almost any cost, you have to stay real with yourself. You have to be fundamentally honest with yourself. It is a terrible irony that a world which is prejudiced puts pressure on people who have a mental illness to be dishonest about themselves, to deny it and so to deny their selves. That is why these stories are such a gift.

Many of us in this book have considered or tried killing ourselves at some point. I think you have to take that as a measure of the pain experienced. The simplest measure, really. And of course, Alasdair finally took that way. When I think about him now I wish to God there had been some other way for him, because he was one of the most courageous people I have ever met.

I heard about his death when I was in Dunedin doing interviews and was so very angry with him. I couldn't believe it had happened. It was only a few weeks after I had seen him so strong. But the point for me about Alasdair's death is that I believe that ultimately we all have the right to say, *This is enough.*

So I'm not angry with him any more. But I am terribly, terribly sad. I miss him. And I will miss him at the book launch. I will miss his face, and his hat and Motley. I will miss his strength.

It was the kind of strength which made me want to do this work and I saw that same strength in all the others in this book. I met some remarkable people during the last two years, people full of hope, determination and creativity.

I finish this work amazed by the ability of human beings to overcome adversity and discover new life.

Gathering and Presenting the Stories

Context defines content and content determines presentation.

Context and Content

My friend Betty Munnoch taught me years ago, that context defines content. We were both students at Edinburgh and used to study together. Before we began a discussion, Betty would always ask me, 'Now when was it written? What was going in the country at that time? What about the politics? What was the economy like? And what about the author, what do we know about the author?' That was one of the most valuable lessons I ever had.

Since then, I have never wanted to separate process from content. That is why I believe it's important to know the process of producing these stories.

The first aim of this work was to produce a book of stories about how people deal successfully with mental illness. The underlying purpose was to produce a document which would help to counter discrimination against people with experience of mental illness.

For me, inevitably, a secondary aim was to understand what it really means to deal successfully with mental illness. What is involved? What lessons can be learned from what people say? Is there something *I* can learn from this which will make my work as a Commissioner better? What will it teach me personally as well?

In a sense, this was also research. This very special kind of writing and research has a fascinating methodology. It's a process of continuous evolution. Because it moves through stages of interview and discussion, transcript, draft story and discussion, final story and discussion, there are opportunities for insights to emerge all the time. Meaning develops as the work progresses.

There was no 'grand' design to this book. I just decided it had to be written and then it just seemed to happen. However, I had written a similar book some years ago and for that I developed a methodology which served me well again.[1]

The people who told me their stories came from all around the country and were not chosen in any systematic way. Some people had heard I was planning this book and asked to be in it. Others were approached directly or by other people. Everyone had the choice of being identified or being anonymous, and I also made it clear that they could drop out at any part of the process, prior to publication.

The initial interviews (which were recorded) were carried out over a period of two years, so the understandings I got about how people deal with mental illness filtered in slowly. And of course they became integrated with and informed by other parts of my experience – both in the present and historically.

In trying to really *hear* people's stories, I had many more advantages than anyone reading this book. For a start, I spent quite a lot of time with most of the people. Some of them I already knew, others I came to know during the past two years. I also heard much fuller versions of their stories – some of the transcripts were over forty pages long. I also heard things which people did not want to be recorded and the things that were recorded which they didn't want to go into the written story. I also heard parts of the story told again in more expansive ways during the second interviews. All of these versions of their stories contributed to my understanding.

When people told me their story, I also watched their faces as they talked to me. I heard the silences in their stories, the inflections in their voices, and the things they repeated in different ways – saying, in effect, 'now this bit is *really* important'. I heard the pauses and the emphases and the tone in which they said things – the moments of wry irony, the sadness, the anger, the relief. Most important of all, I had the opportunity to *relate* to the people. This is the most central gift in understanding. Relating our story is a way we can relate – make a relationship – with someone else.

I try to find *relation points* in an interview. The relation points are what make or break an interview. The best interviews are those in which there are several relation points, because that's where insights begin. It's through the relation points that I understand what somebody is saying, and gain wisdom rather than just information. In this kind of research, I'm not just trying to get facts and information, I'm trying to understand, and so the whole point is that I learn **through** – learn through absorption, learn through my own experience of their experience – learn through insight.

Such interviews are often intimate, and this is one of the reasons why they are so demanding. There's no such thing as going in and being bland and unaffected. Of course some of the relation points are quite painful for me, quite difficult at times. In every case, I was touched by the interview.

In most cases about a year went by before I began to draft the stories. Partly this was because of other work commitments, but in this kind of work, it is important to let time do its job as well. The time lag served two really important purposes. First, it gave people longer to consider whether they really wanted to go ahead with the book. Second, it gave me time to think.

I said earlier that a secondary aim of this work was to understand what it really means to deal successfully with mental illness. The greatest challenge in this kind of work is to tolerate ambiguity and wait for understanding to emerge rather than to try to impose it. Patterns have to be allowed to emerge rather than be 'extracted from data'. It is uncomfortable not to understand things, and tempting to impose clarification, but in this kind of work, solutions cannot be forced.

This analysis is about *being* not *doing*, so that I can absorb the stories I hear and make sense of the worlds of the people I meet. Waiting is part of this analysis. It allows ideas to mature. It is important to take the time to make *connections* between what different people say. It calls for times of stillness. The more I gnaw away at some things, the less I see, and the more I might change them from what they actually are. I have to find a balance between absorption and distance, going in closely, trying to hear and use the language, then standing away, holding onto ambiguity until resolution comes through insight. (I described this process, which I called 'the intuitive analysis' in greater detail in an earlier work.)[2]

The stories were produced during a very intensive twelve week period when I travelled around New Zealand and met people again. These interviews were usually much longer than the first interview, as we now worked together to discuss and finalise their story.

Before each meeting, I cast a draft story by editing the person's transcript. (Every interview had been typed up into a verbatim transcript and checked for accuracy.) The rule I used was that I could delete and move, but not add any words. I chose the most crucial/eloquent/expressive/lucid/articulate parts of the person's story. This was a very subjective process and I saw the results as very much a *first* draft.

I sent the draft story and a full copy of the transcript to the person to make sure I hadn't left out things they really wanted in, and to let them remove or change anything. Then, about a week later, I visited them and we worked on the draft together (directly on the computer) until we arrived at a final version. I aim for 'close-to-spoken language', and at this stage we also tightened the language slightly. After this meeting, I posted two copies of the 'final story' a few days later and asked them to check it and discuss it again with me if necessary, and then give me written approval for publication.

Content and Presentation

The Mental Health Commission produces many documents; usually they are about service provision and are in the form of reports, discussion papers, or newsletters, and mainly for people who work in the mental health sector. The work of the Anti Discrimination Action Plan Team is slightly different because its main task is to challenge assumptions and change ideas about the understanding of mental illness.

This means we have to present our material in ways which encourage people to look at the contents in a *new way*. This is why our 'strategic plan' for reducing discrimination was presented in the form of a map and travel guide.[3] We wanted people to see as well as read that change is a process, not an event. And it usually requires the mind to make a journey. We also wanted to emphasise that social change requires many different journeys, and many different travellers.

At the time we were preparing that document, a few people were concerned because our ideas of presentation didn't conform to the usual style of government reports. We knew, however, that we needed to be creative if we were to communicate our ideas.

'A Gift of Stories' also challenges some traditional ideas. People who have experienced mental illness themselves say what *they* think about mental illness and how to deal with it. For some readers, who are only used to considering what health professionals think, some of the ideas here might be quite a shock. Even more challenging, the information is not given as principles or 'best practice notes', it is given in stories.

So once again, we needed to find a form of presentation which would signal that something different is being said here. That is why the appearance of this document is different from usual government reports, because its *content* is different, and is intimately related to the innovation this project demanded.

One of the purposes of this book is to show that not only does mental illness affect all kinds of people but that people with mental illness have all kinds of facets to their lives. That is why there are pictures throughout the book. I took photographs of each person and of things that are important to them, for example their pictures, poems, artwork, photos of them as a child, certificates about seamanship or social work, marathon achievements, and others. These images are there to remind you that these are real people speaking, who have everyday lives. The 'word-stories' are about the person's experience of mental illness, but the 'picture-stories' are simply about the person. Finally, we want it to be known that mental illness can also be a gift. Moreover, many of the contributors are artists of various kinds. This is why we wanted the book to be beautiful.

Once again, it is possible that some people will find the presentation of this book disturbingly unusual. It is always disturbing to be at the edge of change. It is an extremely uncomfortable place to be and people who are there constantly have to find the courage to stay there. They have to justify what they do, they have to stick to their principles in the face of challenge, and finally they have simply to disregard the seductive trap of the argument that 'safety lies in being the same'.

To make a difference, we need to act differently – but not simply for the sake of being different. There has to be a fundamental logic as to why and how we need to be different. It is only by being at the edge of change that the Mental Health Commission will make a difference – which is what we have committed ourselves to doing.

Notes

1 *Straight to the Point. See* Leibrich, above. This book won the Legal Research Foundation special prize in 1994 and has been used for teaching methodology in various universities.
2 *Ibid.*
3 *A travel guide for people on the journeys towards equality, respect and rights for people who experience mental illness.* Mental Health Commission, Wellington, 1999.

Some Words of Thanks

When you are in the last stages of creating a book, it is easy to forget about all the people who have helped at the various stages, because at the end, only the writing seems important. But it is the experiences on the way which finally lead to publication.

First of all, I want to thank my colleagues at the Mental Health Commission who have made so many contributions to this work – in sharing ideas and commitment. This book could not have been produced without the support of all of them.

Inevitably, in a workplace, there are some people with whom you work more closely than others and so in particular, I want to thank my fellow Commissioners Barbara Disley and Bob Henare, with whom it is a privilege to work; the members of the Anti Discrimination Action Plan Team – Tessa Thompson and Mary O'Hagan, and earlier on, Margaret Thompson – for it is the work of that team which continues to inspire me and which ultimately led to the creation of this book; Joy Cooper and Wayne Miles for sharing their extensive and deep knowledge of the mental health system; our kaumatua Denis Simpson, and Fuimaono Karl Pulotu-Endemann for helping me understand differ-

ent cultures, and finally, Leah Sorenson, my PA, for looking after me with a brilliant combination of organisational skills and personal care.

I couldn't even have imagined doing this book without Lynne Rice and Kathy Steinmetz, who typed all the transcriptions. We have worked as a team on an earlier book and I just knew things would be okay if we could work as a team on this one, too. I am deeply grateful for their professionalism and their warmth and humour. And I knew, too, that if I had David Guerin's eye on the text as I was editing, I would commit no major crime! So I am very thankful for his work during my editing of the stories. And, as always, for the insight he brings to the underlying ideas.

I have two special readers for anything I write. They are my husband, Doug Harvie, and my very dear friend, Betty Munnoch. They are my 'wise' people. Once again I have been able to have them with me on this journey all the way. We go a long way back – they know me and my foibles and they are two people I can trust to say when I'm off course.

Doug is a mathematician and a kind of gentle sceptic. But also a great believer in humanity. His in-

put and personal support has been invaluable to me. He has not only had to read the book as I was putting it together, but also cook the meals – an added bonus!

Betty and I have shared a longstanding love of literature from when we were students at Edinburgh University together thirty years ago. She has been my mentor and my 'Virgil' for many years, leading me through many times of Purgatory and getting me safely to the other side. We have lived on different sides of the world all these years, but that has never stopped our flow of amazing communication.

Other friends have played a major role in this book, too – listening to me rave on, talking through the concepts, and basically just being understanding. It is hard to select one or two to mention but I must. I want to thank Kim Saffron, especially for her wit and reason and kindness; Ruth Brown and Wendy Norman who have born the brunt of my delights and despairs during our early morning beach walks over the last few months and never wavered in their support of me; and Kathy Ansin and Barbara Coad for helping me keep going.

During the last few days of getting the book ready for print, my brother Tony Halstead visited me from England. His comments and insight into what I personally was trying to say in this book were invaluable.

There are many kinds of support I am grateful for. Ruth Manchester has guided me through this work and has helped me with some tough decisions during my work as a Commissioner. And I thank my 'shooting the breeze' friends at Café Palms, where I learn so much, especially Roger Hewitson and Ian Dennis.

Now I come to Wendy Harrex, the publisher. I have worked with Wendy before as well and knew that when she took 'my baby' from me, I could feel sure that it would be looked after properly – and even loved.

I was very lucky the day I met Susie Crooks. Not only did she give me a fantastic story for the book, but she also agreed to take on the role of designer. She had said to me one day 'You know, this book will be a täonga – a treasure. And it should look like one too!' I knew that if I put that work in her hands, then it would. Anneloes Douglas was a University of Otago design student on a placement with Wendy Harrex at the time this book was being published and she interpreted Susie's ideas beautifully in her layout of the chapter openings and cover. Fiona Moffat of the University of Otago Press has worked on the text pages and production.

Most of all though, I want to thank the contributors to this book. Each of them has given not only to the project, but also to me personally. I have enjoyed meeting and getting to know every one of them. I have been allowed into other worlds and welcomed there. What more could I have asked for?

Julie Leibrich
Raumati, August, 1999